BEHIND CLOSED DOORS

Gender, Sexuality, and Touch in the Doctor/Patient Relationship

Angelica Redleaf
with Susan A. Baird

AUBURN HOUSE
Westport, Connecticut • London

Library of Congress Cataloging-in-Publication Data

Redleaf, Angelica, 1946–
   Behind closed doors : gender, sexuality, and touch in the
doctor/patient relationship / Angelica Redleaf, with Susan A. Baird.
      p.   cm.
   Includes bibliographical references and index.
   ISBN 0–86569–285–8 (alk. paper)
   1. Physician and patient.   2. Sex (Psychology)   3. Touch—
Psychological aspects.   4. Defensive medicine.   I. Baird, Susan
A., 1961– . II. Title.
   R727.3.R4   1998
   610.69′6—dc21   97–32947

British Library Cataloguing in Publication Data is available.

Library of Congress Catalog Card Number: 97–32947
ISBN: 0–86569–285–8

First published in 1998

Auburn House, 88 Post Road West, Westport, CT 06881
An imprint of Greenwood Publishing Group, Inc.

Printed in the United States of America

The paper used in this book complies with the
Permanent Paper Standard issued by the National
Information Standards Organization (Z39.48–1984).

10 9 8 7 6 5 4 3 2

Copyright Acknowledgments

The author and publisher gratefully acknowledge permisison to use quotations and extracts from Ben Benjamin: *Massage and Bodywork with Survivors of Abuse*, Medford, MA: Ben Benjamin, p. 73, 1995; Ben Benjamin and Angelica Redleaf: "Risk Factor Analysis," The Association for Chiropractic Excellence, Inc., pp. 1–6, 1995; Ben Benjamin and Angelica Redleaf: "Sexual Misconduct Risk Factor Analysis: Are You at Risk?" The Association for Chiropractic Excellence, Inc., 1–7, 1996; Ben Benjamin and Angelica Redleaf: "Determine Your Risk Factor: Sexual Misconduct" and "Five-Minute Self Exam," *Chiropractic Economics* 38(6):46–48, 1996; Angelica Redleaf and Susan Baird: "ACE Patient Protection Protocol," The Association for Chiropractic Excellence, Inc., pp. 22–28, 1996.

Contents

PART II   Sexual Misconduct

Preface

What goes on behind closed doors in a doctor's office? All sorts of things—and most of them, certainly, occur for the good of the patient. But some of the things that go on in a doctor's office do the patient no good at all.

If we were not sexual beings, this book would not be necessary. But we are. Moreover, we live in a society that is obsessed with sex and sexuality, yet has very little understanding of how they affect men and women, doctors and patients. Clearly, there are doctors who knowingly hurt their patients, and we'll take a look at why they do so. It is my belief, however, that the vast majority of the harm done to patients is not intended.

Most doctors—indeed, most health-care professionals—have only good intentions. But good intentions are not enough. We must ask ourselves, do we know what effects our attitudes and our behaviors have on our patients? Most of us don't—and we need to find out. Understanding how our patients perceive us and how they experience our actions is the first step in a process that can enable us to go beyond good intentions, to good results.

This book's purpose is two-fold: to alert doctors to their own behaviors and attitudes, and to the ways in which they may inadvertently cause harm to their patients; and to provide doctors with new skills that will allow them to care for their patients more safely, with less risk to both doctor and patient.

In the pages ahead, we'll examine the power dynamics between doctor and patient; the elusive issue of patient consent; and the effect of gender, sexuality and touch on the doctor/patient relationship. We'll offer several exercises to help doctors explore their own attitudes toward these seldom-discussed topics.

We'll discuss the special concerns of caring for patients who have previously been abused, and for all patients, so that everyone will feel safe and properly cared for.

Finally, we'll present a blueprint for a multi-stage program of personal and professional development, for improving doctor/patient communication and creating a health care environment that is safer and more fulfilling for both doctor and patient.

It is my hope that this book will raise awareness of several issues in practice that are potentially volatile, yet are hidden beneath the surface. This book, I hope, will help many more doctors to see beneath that surface. This book is not intended to cover every aspect of these issues, nor to provide a solution for every conceivable situation, but it is a beginning. Learning about sexual misconduct, and about doctor behavior in general, is like peeling an onion. As one layer is peeled away, another appears.

In closing, I would like to offer sincere thanks to the following people who encouraged us, helped and advised us, and were instrumental in making this book a reality:

My family: my mother Edith, my grandmother Mia, Robert, Friedl, Gerda, Alice, George, Dennis, Ronnie, Kristen, and Eric.

My surrogate family: Natalie Redleaf, Gil Redleaf, Joan, Ben, Fred and Greg Kingsbury, and Leone and Wayne Pippin.

The people who believed in me, even when I didn't: Judge Haiganush Bedrosian, Julia Deisler, Candice Dunn, Debra Duxbury, Cambrea Ezekiel, Ellen Gittleman, Mariah Martin, Laurie Moriarty, Michelle Morra, Judith Nutkis, Kathleen O'Sullivan, Joe Pagana, Gwenneth Rae, Ed.D., Carol Ricci, Donna Rogers, Robin Romeo, Leya Tadesse, Donna Vagshenian, Gloria Vignone, and Jan Wilson.

My colleagues: Mark A. Davini, Maureen Flammer, Beth Goulding, Victoria Malchar, Lawrence Markson, Robert Quigley, Roger Redleaf, Michael Rogers, Vernon Temple, and Michael J. Zola, all of whom are doctors of chiropractic, and Marsha Woolf, N.D., licensed acupuncturist.

My business associates Al Gemma, Esq., and Frank Mansella, CPA.

My patients, who over the years have trusted me with their health, their bodies, and, at times, their souls.

Those who specifically helped with this book: My editor and co-writer Susan Baird; Linda Handel, who put us in touch with Anne Waterman; Anne Waterman, through whose efforts we found a publisher; Nita Romer, at Greenwood Publishing Group, who decided to accept our book for publication; Julie Cullen, our production editor; the people who assisted us by providing important information, reviewing the manuscript, or both, especially Ben Benjamin, Ph.D., John C. Gonsiorek, Ph.D., Larry Markson, D.C., Jeanette Hofstee Milgrom, Peter Rutter, M.D., and Gary R. Schoener, M.A.; and those doctors and patients who were willing to share with us their personal experiences with sexual misconduct and unprofessional behavior.

And those who inspired me: Gloria Steinem (thank you for lunch!), Estelle Disch, Ph.D., Carol Gilligan, Ph.D., the Stone Center at Wellesley College, and the Walk-In Counseling Center in Minneapolis, Minn.

I also would like to take this opportunity to acknowledge the efforts of

Canada, and in particular, of the province of Ontario, which has led the way in promoting ethical and safe health-care. Throughout this book, specific mention and quotes will cite Ontario's actions.

Angelica Redleaf, D.C.

PART I

Gender, Sexuality, and Touch

A man and a woman who close the door behind them to have a private meeting find themselves in a situation in which sex is possible—as do two women and two men if they are gay.

—*Deborah Tannen,*
"Talking from 9 to 5," 1994

— *1* —

Gender

GENDER: the fact or condition of being a male or a female human being, esp. with regard to how this affects or determines a person's self-image, social status, goals, etc.

Webster's New World Dictionary,
Third College Edition, 1994

Just what is gender and how does it affect us? How does gender affect people in other cultures? What is the impact of gender on the health-care relationship? These are the questions on which this chapter will focus.

GENDER AND CULTURE

Our Gendered World

The first thing a doctor says about a newborn child is "It's a boy!" or "It's a girl!" The first thing people ask about a young child is its gender. And gender is the first consideration in selecting infants' clothing, much of which is manufactured in gender-specific baby blue or baby pink.

We, in our society, rarely write, speak or think about someone without acknowledging or considering his or her gender. Take heed, the next time you run across a description of someone in an article or a book: One of the first things described, if not *the* first, will be whether that person is male or female. Notice, the next time someone is being described to you: Is femaleness or maleness among the first attributes listed? And when you describe an individual, is gender one of the most important of the attributes you list?

Gender is often the most important piece of information upon which we base our decisions and assumptions. Yet psychologists say we all have masculine and feminine aspects to our personalities. Some of us, regardless of gender, will exhibit more characteristics that are considered male; others will exhibit more female characteristics. Human characteristics would be a better way to describe them, as these character traits know no gender boundaries.

The Interaction of Language and Culture

How we think is shaped in part by the language we speak. All languages have a profound effect on those who speak them. Language structures the way in which its speakers see the world, and the English language is no exception. For example, English gives us no pronoun to refer to an individual of unspecified gender. We have only he, she, or it—and to refer to a person as "it" is to be intentionally, unspeakably rude. "He or she," "he/she," and "s/he" are some of the awkward alternatives that have been proposed. English does at least have the non-gender-specific plurals "we" and "they." The Latinate tongues do not provide such an option.

But gender does not shape every language as strongly as it does the European tongues.

Thomson Highway, a Cree Indian who spoke about his culture and language at a 1994 conference in Ontario, Canada, explained that the Cree don't separate the world into male and female as we do. Instead, their language divides the world into animate and inanimate. Highway said that the people in his culture don't think twice about male housewives or female breadwinners or same-gender relationships, because the people who exhibit such behaviors are not breaking traditional roles or violating stereotypes. They are simply at the less-populated end of a wide spectrum of behavior, all of which is acceptable. Their differences are cherished, rather than disparaged.[1]

In the Swahili language, the world is divided into other sorts of categories: round objects, which include their houses; pointed objects, which include their weapons and some of their cooking tools; things that are carried, which include bags, bedding, and babies; and people. Not male and female people, just people.

In Western society, we divide our world into masculine and feminine. It is difficult to think of a person without first thinking of his or her gender. That's partly a function of our languages and partly a function of the concepts that our society emphasizes. If we divided our world differently, we would see it differently. Very few people are able to conceptualize something for which they have no words. Take snow, for instance.

The Inuit people (the Eskimos) are said to have forty-four words for snow. Snow, for them, is vital, and so the different kinds of snow need to be readily differentiated. They must distinguish light, powdery snow, for instance, from deep, crusted-over snow that may cave in dangerously underfoot. When they look at snow, they see subtleties that most of us never notice, unless snow is very important to us. When skiers look at snow, they may see packed powder (light, dry snow that has been compressed by time or by trail-grooming equipment) or corn snow (snow that has melted and refrozen into coarse clumps). When most people look at snow, they see just snow. Or perhaps they see that it's time to get out the snow shovel, or to book a cruise to the Caribbean.

The specific language a person uses may affect even the development of the brain. Native speakers of Japanese and English, for instance, think about things very differently. (They have to, because their languages are constructed very differently. For instance, Japanese has nothing quite the same as our notion of a verb.) And they use different regions of the cerebral cortex to do it.

GENDER ROLES IN WESTERN SOCIETY

Like language, our cultural or ethnic background profoundly affects how we see our world. These factors shape the way we think and feel about males and females. We may wish to believe that we, alone, have formed our ideas about gender—but we have not done this in a vacuum. The conclusions that we reach are inescapably affected by the culture in which we were raised and within which we live. Contributing to this ongoing process of acculturation are the news and entertainment media, which have bombarded us with umpteen messages about what are and are not ideal male and female behaviors and attributes. And, as we all know, these ''ideal'' and ''not ideal'' attributes change from generation to generation.

Twentieth Century Icons

Here are some cultural icons from the last few generations. Who else comes to mind? Which of these people do you look up to? Which ones are like you?

Erroll Flynn	In movie after movie, his sexy swashbuckler—a rogue who was always a gentlemen with the ladies—let men and women dream of having their romance and adventure, and security, too.
Mae West	''Come on up and see me some time'' outlaw babe—smart, sophisticated, bad only because she liked sex; ''if you can't be good, be good at it.''
Katharine Hepburn	Quiet rebel . . . loved anyway; untraditional beauty.
Audrey Hepburn	Spunky yet demure; always perfectly polished.
Fred Astaire	Debonair dancer of the Silver Screen.
Ginger Rogers	Astaire's sometime co-star and dance partner, this glamorous actress is famously described as having done everything that he did, ''but backwards and in high heels.''
Jimmy Stewart	The original sensitive guy.
Rock Hudson	To-die-for hunk who, in real life, turned out to prefer gentlemen.
Doris Day	Spunky girl next door.
John Wayne	Home on the range.
Donna Reed	Home at the range.
Prince Rainier and Princess Grace	Cinderella tale come true, for once, except that this Cinderella (actress Grace Kelly) came from a prominent upper-class family.

Richard Burton and Elizabeth Taylor	These two abided by the gender roles, but not the sexual mores, of their time. When he dumped his family to be with her, she got the bad name. But times change. Now they're both known as passionate, outrageous, brilliant stars.
John F. Kennedy and Jacqueline Kennedy Onassis	As the President and First Lady who presided over "Camelot," they were lauded as the ideal couple. She stood by her man, despite the philandering that became public knowledge only after his death. Her reward was general condemnation when, rather than remaining the eternal widow, she went on with her life and married again. The public forgave her, but it took decades.
Elvis Presley	Shook his hips, and shook up America; but his shocking pelvic gyrations look pretty tame, by today's standards.
Marilyn Monroe and James Dean	Bad, but good at it—and both paid the ultimate price.
Tina Turner and Ike	For years, she stood by her man, even though he exploited and beat her. He said she'd be nothing without him. Then she told him to take a hike—and got a bigger, better life and career.
Ward and June Cleaver, of *Leave it to Beaver*	Asexual mainstream role models of the 1960s. He brings in the bacon, she cooks it. He dispenses advice, she dispenses Band-Aids. He solves the big problems at home, she vacuums the rug.
Burt Reynolds and Dolly Parton	Unabashed mainstream sex symbols—but she just *looks* sexy, while he's known for doing something about it.
Mel Gibson	Boyish charmer who's aging gracefully.
Meryl Streep	Speaking of aging gracefully—Streep has shown that, after almost fifty years, older women again can be sexy . . . and they don't have to become outcasts to do it.
Clint Eastwood and Sharon Stone	Sexy and steely; people eat it up in the theaters—and for Clint, in politics, too. But after her cold-blooded role in *Basic Instinct*, how many people would be ready to vote for Sharon Stone?
Tom Hanks	Boyish, bashful, endearing. The 1990s' answer to Jimmy Stewart, Hanks has the charm but not the sex appeal.
Sigourney Weaver	The star of the *Alien* movies, and others, she displays confidence, competence, and great pecs as she races through one hair-breadth escape after another, with nary a teetering high heel. She may be the first female action hero whose role was meant to be taken seriously.
Antonio Banderas	Sexy man, strong actor, and possible heir to Erroll Flynn—but neither he nor his female co-stars get quite so carried away.
Meg Tilly	Lovely, graceful, and iron-willed, she is no wilting lily.
Leonardo DiCaprio	To his hordes of adoring fans, this slender young star is the epitome of the teddy-bear-like teen idol: "more chipper than smoldering, too boyish to be androgynous but too androgenous to be sexy in any threatening, carnal, actual sort of way."[2]

These days, it seems, the bad boys aren't as bad as they used to be—or, if they are, they aren't accepted in polite society. And these days, the good girls get to have a lot more fun. What other changes do you see in the people we elevate to icon status, as we flow from the era of Erroll Flynn to Antonio Banderas, and from Mae West to Meg Tilly, or even Madonna?

Gender-Role Rebels

Musicians and other rebels spurred heated controversy in the 1960s and 1970s—as they have since time immemorial—with hairdos, or clothing, or makeup that did not fit that era's image of men or women.

In the 1980s, a group of public figures began to emerge who went even further in their refusal to conform to traditional roles. They are blurring the lines our culture has drawn to distinguish between men and women. Who else can you think of? Has your perspective changed?

Michael Jackson	This is one attempt to move beyond gender limitations, but the overall effect is of asexuality gone awry. It is no accident that he has been most popular with kids who haven't hit puberty.
Richard Simmons	Brave enough to be himself, this high-voiced mild-mannered man looks like a "before" picture, succeeds as a fitness guru.
Madonna	Blatantly omnivorous. A competent musician who has made her real career of breaking all the rules and playing all the roles.
The former Prince	Macho man in Lycra and lace, he refuses to be bound by societal conventions—including the prerequisite of a pronounceable name.
Mariel Hemingway	Deliberately ambiguous.
Greg Louganis	Olympic diver who makes the agonizing decision to come out of the closet as a gay man, with HIV, and initially is condemned.
k.d. lang	Country music star who raises eyebrows but few tempers with transgender stunts like the magazine cover on which she is pictured in a barber's chair getting a shave from a supermodel.
Ellen DeGeneres	Lesbian sitcom star who comes out on prime time, in one of the most hyped shows in history, playing a bookstore manager who realizes that she is a lesbian.
Melissa Etheridge	Successful musician comes out of the closet and stays successful; then, she and her partner succeed in making lesbian motherhood as wholesome as apple pie.
Rocky Horror Picture Show	The cult classic B-movie of the 1970s whose star plays a "transsexual Transylvanian."
Priscilla, Queen of the Desert	Low-budget Australian film, about the adventures of three drag queens cruising the Outback, was a surprise U.S. success.
To Wong Foo, With Love	Mainstream American film, made after *Priscilla*'s success, traces the adventures of three drag queens cruising the Midwest. (Is there an echo?) Stars three very successful, very macho actors.
The Birdcage	*Les Cages aux Folles*, the classic French art film about an outrageous, theatrical, cross-dressing gay couple and their son, also goes mainstream—with the unabashedly heterosexual comic actor Robin Williams in the starring role.

Images of Health Professionals

Our culture's images of health professionals also have changed through the generations. Are you like any of these?

Florence Nightingale	A real-life heroine who left behind a life of luxury for a career as a nurse, helping to make nursing almost respectable. But she also came to symbolize a willingness to sacrifice everything to serve.
Marcus Welby, M.D.	An elderly general practitioner, the fictional doctor was fatherly, usually right, always compassionate, and he made house calls.
Dr. Steven Kiley, of *Marcus Welby, M.D.*	Welby's suave young motorcycle-riding sidekick, he was added to update the show. He flirted with all the nurses and cute female patients. Boy, would he be in trouble today!
Dr. Kildare	Cool, crisp, professional, and always right, the title character was a modern, hospital-based practitioner who saved lives without ever creasing his white coat, or his detachment. A true product of the era of wonder drugs. Did he even *have* a first name?
Dr. "Hawkeye" Pierce, of *M*A*S*H*	A besotted, skirt-chasing surgical genius, this lead character in the popular movie and television series was rebellious and discontented because he had been drafted to patch up soldiers fighting a war he didn't believe in (the Korean). But he was still a sensitive guy. All was forgiven because he was so highly skilled.
Major Margaret "Hotlips" Houlihan, R.N., of *M*A*S*H*	Military officer and nurse, so the writers touched on all the stereotypes, making her bossy, butch, and hard as nails, but also beautiful, sexy, and incredibly sex-starved—a trait she shared with most of the *M*A*S*H* characters. All that, and a heart of gold, too.
Dr. Beverly Crusher, of *Star Trek: The Next Generation*	Single mother (respectably widowed) and chief medical officer of a starship the size of a small city, this character was one of the first female doctors to be prominently featured on prime-time television.
Dr. Kate Austin, of *Chicago Hope*	A talented cardiothoracic surgeon—and another single mother —who made television history, in the spring of 1996, when her character was named the hospital's new chief of surgery. But, perhaps reflecting a lingering ambivalence toward women in positions of authority, her hold on that position is tenuous: She since has been removed as chief of surgery, and later reinstated.

Notice how the depictions of doctors and nurses have changed? Doctors used to be seen as infallible, inhuman, and mostly male, and nurses as either serious and sacrificing or sex-starved and self-serving. We've come a long way!

Accepted Gender Roles

In their book *Megatrends for Women*, authors Patricia Aburdene and John Naisbitt list some of the traits our society looks for in each gender (they draw their list from an analysis of masculine and feminine stereotypes by Merlin

Table 1.1
Innate Gender Traits

Men	Women
more upper-body strength and wider shoulders, giving better leverage and weight-lifting ability, proportionally	wider hips and lower center of gravity, giving better balance and ability to carry more weight, proportionally
lesser tolerance for pain	more tolerance for pain
deeper voices	higher voices
better tolerance for loud noises	better hearing, especially of high-pitched sounds (such as a baby's cry)
sounder sleepers/need less sleep	lighter sleepers/need more sleep
need less sleep	need more sleep
on average, after age 12, are larger and stronger than females	on average, until age 10 or 12, are larger and stronger than males
more lean muscle mass, proportionally	less lean muscle mass, proportionally
less tendency to accumulate body fat, but what does build up is more likely to be high-risk, fat use abdominal fat	greater tendency to accumulate body fat, but more of that is low-risk, slow-burning peripheral ''famine'' fat
faster metabolisms	slower metabolisms
faster runners/swimmers over short to marathon distances	may have biological advantage in long-distance swimming and ultra-marathon land races
higher frequency of genetic defects	have stronger immune systems
born in greater numbers	live longer, on average
may have better spatial abilities	may have better communication abilities
better peripheral circulation; more comfortable in extreme heat or cold	circulation gives higher priority to internal organs; survive longer in extreme heat or cold
ejaculate, sire children	menstruate, bear children
later physical and sexual maturation; later onset of infertility	earlier physical maturation; earlier onset of infertility

Stone, author of *When God Was a Woman*). Their conclusions:

[T]here are positive traits on both lists. On the feminine list are the most important traits for human interaction. And although the masculine list appears outer-directed and success-oriented, many of the characteristics required at the very *top* levels of leadership appear on the female list. What leader can afford to sacrifice cooperation, fail at nurturing and supporting or ignore the flash of intuition where every piece of data comes together? . . . The point is: *successful human beings possess a combination of masculine and feminine traits.* The most creative are a hybrid of supposedly conflicting characteristics: competitive and compassionate; goal-oriented and nurturing; intuitive and risk taking. Cardboard, one-dimensional females and males alike are doomed to failure.[3]

We all know people of one gender who exhibit some or even many traits of the other gender. We might do better to speak about general tendencies, or even a continuum of traits shared by both genders. Imagine what it would be like to be accepted unconditionally, regardless of the gender-role traits that we exhibit.

GENDER TRAITS

Innate Traits. Are there traits innate to each gender? There seem to be a few, but not nearly so many as was once thought. Most experts currently agree on the traits listed in Table 1.1, above.

Men are generally considered to have a greater tendency toward aggression, but this tendency has not been quantified, or even proven. What is known is that cultural contributors to this behavior are considerably more important, on average, than any biological bias. Both genders experience periodic fluctuations in hormones that are known to affect their moods and levels of aggression; in women, these fluctuations are related to the monthly menstrual cycle, whereas in men, these fluctuations are more rapid and less regular.

Margaret Mead, in her anthropological examinations of the aboriginal peoples of Samoa, uncovered some interesting data regarding aggression and socialization: Among the Arapesh, both men and women were quiet and nurturing; they were "unaggressive and non-initiatory, non-competitive and responsive, warm, docile and trusting." Among the Mundugumore, both men and women were "violent, competitive, aggressively sexed . . . delighting in display, in action, in fighting." Among the Tchambuli, women were expected to be impersonal, aggressive, and reliable, whereas men were expected to be warm, docile, and emotionally dependent.[4]

The discovery of such significant variations from Western expectations regarding gender and aggression, in societies coexisting in such proximity to one another, demonstrates the remarkable extent to which aggression and other gender-linked traits can be determined by society, rather than by biology.

Imposed Traits. The traits in Table 1.2 reflect differences between men and women that are suspected of being due, all or in part, to social conditioning.

Table 1.2
Socially Imposed Gender Traits

Men	Women
take more risks	earlier mental, emotional maturation
more active	more deft and precise
more aggressive	more docile and obedient
less emotional, less sensitive to the emotions of others	better communicators of emotional information, even in early childhood

The Influence of Individuality. It is important to remember that, even though some tendencies are considered to be innate to each gender, those traits vary a great deal more *within* each gender than *between* the genders. Men as a group are stronger than women as a group, but some women are far stronger than the average man; women as a group live longer than men as a group, but some men live to 100 or beyond—decades longer than the average woman.

EVOLUTIONARY INSIGHTS

In his book *Men in Groups*, Lionel Tiger puts forward the hypothesis that male bonding and dominance behaviors are phenomena with biological roots. "My proposition is that specialization for hunting widened the gap between the *behaviour* of males and females. It favoured those 'genetic packages' which arranged matters so that males hunted co-operatively in groups while females engaged in maternal and some gathering activity. Not only were there organic changes in perception, brain size, posture, hand formation, locomotion, etc., but there were also social structural changes."[5]

Knowledge of the cultural evolution of gender roles may help us to figure out our starting points, but it does little to help us to establish our roles in the modern world; we are, after all, more than just "the naked ape."[6] We are not about to abandon our society, our culture, our art, medicine and technology for a life as bare-skinned beasts scavenging in the forest. So, why should we follow our furry cousins, as some have argued, in our relationships between genders? "Anatomy is destiny," Sigmund Freud declared,[7] but developmental psychologists and biologists now are replying with a resounding "Not so."

THE EFFECTS OF SOCIALIZATION

> 'Tis education forms the common mind, Just as the twig is bent, the tree's inclined.
>
> —*Alexander Pope,*
> *"Eloise to Abelard," 1717*

Nature vs. Nurture

For much of this century, the war has raged over nature vs. nurture. The biologists declared that nature—that is, genetics, hormonal impulses, and encoded instincts—created and controlled our patterns of behavior. The behavioralists declared that nurture—that is, socialization—deserved almost exclusive credit for our behavior. Although the final verdict is not in, it has nonetheless become clear that both factors are important. The ways in which we socialize our boys and girls is as important as, or perhaps more important than, any innate gender differences. So, what behaviors are we teaching our children?

Boys' message: "Snips and snails, and puppy dogs' tails, that's what little boys are made of."

Girls' message: "Sugar and spice, and everything nice, that's what little girls are made of."

Infancy: The Hand that Rocks the Cradle. From infancy, parents, teachers and the rest of our society tend to encourage boys to be active and girls to be still. They encourage boys to be aggressive and girls to be compliant. They encourage boys to suppress emotion and girls to express it. When a young baby is active, people who have been told that the child is a boy are apt to engage it in more active play; if they think it is a girl, they are apt to quiet the baby instead, engaging in soothing behavior. Our cultural indoctrination begins before we come home from the hospital.

Early Childhood: Molding the Mind. "Women's commitment to alliances and consensus is shaped early. Through age 3, girls and boys behave similarly. But at age 4, boys begin to break their dependence on their mother or caretaker. Girls, meanwhile, immerse themselves in intimacy and are trained to be empathic."[8] By the time that children are old enough to engage in active play, clear behavioral differences have already been established between girls and boys. The spoken and unspoken messages to boys are "boys will be boys" and "don't be a crybaby," whereas girls get the messages to "be nice" and "act like a lady." By the time that they reach school, children have internalized these messages and have learned to reinforce them. Boys who appear more dominant are approved and rewarded by their peers, whereas girls are rejected for showing these traits.

Yet the way in which we treat our children has effects that go far beyond indoctrination into gender roles. The care that they receive as infants and toddlers shapes the very development of their brains, in ways that will have a lifelong effect. A child's brain is not fully formed at birth, as we once thought, but is still actively changing for the first few years of life.

It has long been known that a child born with cataracts, or with an eyelid that failed to open, has to be treated at a very early age. The circuits for vision are formed by the age of two; and if they are not used before then, the child will never be able to see. Similar windows of opportunity exist for hard-wiring other sorts of abilities. The ability to distinguish the different sounds used in language, for instance, is now thought to be determined by the age of one year.

By the time that children are old enough to enter most pre-schools, the window of opportunity is closing, not only for vision, but also for emotion, social skills and vocabulary. More skills can be learned later in life, but the hard-wiring that affects the ability to learn is pretty much set—by age two, for emotion and socialization; and by age three for vocabulary. By the time children are old enough for kindergarten, it is generally too late to dramatically affect their ability to reason, and the window of opportunity for motor development is closing. The circuitry that enables us to learn math and logic is pretty much in place by age four. The hard-wiring for motor skills is firming up by age five.

This early experience shapes most of what we consider "gender traits." We now know that we are who we are much earlier than we had thought. Therefore, if we want young people to become fully developed, we need to be aware of this information and apply it as we raise and educate our children.

Reciprocation of emotions also plays a powerful role. Studies show that when a child's emotions are reciprocated, those emotions are, in effect, normalized—that is, they learn that it's okay to feel those emotions. When those emotions are not modeled by another human, however, the child may become passive, incapable of experiencing happiness. Even as adults, having our emotions met with a blank stare, or with emotions very different from our own, can be very confusing and even painful. We can also find ourselves in a panic when we are completely out of sync with our environment.

When children are treated in a soothing manner, the child in later life learns how to soothe himself or herself. This is a good skill for anyone to possess.

Similar principles apply to athletic skills, which must be reinforced before kindergarten, and math and logic skills, which must be internalized by age four.

When there is a great deal of fear in a child's environment, that fear—which can cause an arousal state that prevents other information from coming through—can profoundly affect the child's development. Basically, under extreme stress, normal development is sacrificed in favor of survival. Constant stress in a child's earliest years can impair learning of upper-brain skills such as emotion, socialization and reasoning. It may also create a sort of "learned helplessness" that is extremely difficult to unlearn.

School Daze. Research over the last decade has shown that in co-educational classes, teachers—even female teachers—still give more attention and respect to boys, reward them for asking questions, and get them engaged in debate. Girls are rewarded for sitting still and shutting up. When boys and girls are tested individually, few differences in intellectual performance are seen, but when boys and girls are observed interacting, many differences appear. The result of this passive role is that girls in mixed-gender classrooms tend to lose ground, academically, during their school years.

It should be observed that girls are not the only ones to suffer from this differential treatment: Girls are denied the opportunity to learn to shine in active debate. Boys are denied the opportunity to learn to perform in passive situations. It should also be observed that the differential spills over into many aspects of adult life—something that is true of nonacademic socialization, as well. The competitive and team-play skills taught in school sports, for example—a socialization that girls used to be denied because they were not, until recently, welcomed into team sports—are the model that still prevails in the world of business.

Adolescence: The Terrible Teens. Carol Gilligan, a Harvard University psychologist, has been at the forefront of those studying the internal lives of girls and women. Her research, which has been done in part with colleagues at the Stone Center at Wellesley College in Wellesley, Mass., has yielded some very interesting findings.

For example, Gilligan reports that girls reach a psychological impasse, at about age eleven, upon first encountering the conventions of a male-dominated culture. They suddenly realize that their sharp awareness of intimacy is seen as something of little value, despite the general perception of women as caring and altruistic. Boys and girls tend to have a similar level of self-esteem until the time of puberty. Then, everything changes.

A recent survey by the American Association of University Women supports Gilligan's conclusion that girls (specifically, Caucasian girls, in the AAUW study) suffer a tremendous loss of self-esteem—thirty-one points—between the ages of eight and sixteen.

This drop in self-esteem, combined with classroom training in deferring to their male colleagues, helps to explain why girls and women are more apt to be tentative or even silent in mixed-gender settings such as classrooms, meetings, or the work place.

Young Adulthood: Settling Into Our Roles. By the time we reach young adulthood, our gender roles are clearly defined. Women have been shown their place in our society—and if at some point they should "forget," they are apt to be quickly and perhaps not so gently reminded. Many people still are uncomfortable with men who seem too "feminine." Many people don't like women whom they see as too "masculine." We are so enculturated into our masculine and feminine roles that we may lose sight of where our roles end and we begin.

Mid-Life: A Role of One's Own.

> Youth is the time of getting, middle age of improving, and old age of spending.
>
> *Anne Bradstreet,*
> *"Meditations Divine and Moral," 1664*

As people reach their middle years, some simply become more settled in their ways; but for others, it is a time of change as profound as adolescence. Carl Gustav Jung, the Swiss psychoanalyst, was among the many who noted that at mid-life many people experience a transition, a shift from one way of being to another. It is worth noting that the concept of "middle age" is an ancient one, far predating Anne Bradstreet or even the Middle Ages; it is recognized even in Classical mythology, in the Sphinx's riddle about the ages of man.[9]

Gail Sheehy, in her book *New Passages*, writes of this transition: "It could be called the Meaning Crisis. It is based on a spiritual imperative: The wish to integrate the disparate aspects of ourselves, the hunger for wholeness, the need to know the truth. Women are more likely to develop their rational thinking functions and enjoy extending their powers into a broader arena, while men are often drawn inward, from thinking to feeling."[10]

As men and women reach their middle years, they tend to give more weight to their own opinion of themselves and society, and less to society's opinion of them. They are likely to be less concerned about staying within—or rebelling against—the roles dictated by their gender or social class or profession. And if they feel that something is lacking, or that there is some imbalance, they may attempt to fill the gap in their knowledge, or to right the imbalance.

Regardless of gender, as we reach this stage in life, many of us find ourselves working to build up the traits that we played down in our youth.

PSYCHOLOGICAL DEVELOPMENT

The Male Model: The Independent Man

Experts in the field of psychiatry, including Sigmund Freud and Erik Erikson, have held up one model of "normal" psychological development for everyone: the model of the Independent Man. In this model of development of the self, we begin as totally dependent infants. As we develop a degree of control over our environment, we recognize ourselves as separate entities. During childhood, we gradually increase our "sense of psychological separation." By the time we reach adulthood, it is expected that we will have become completely independent, autonomous beings, with full self-control.

An important question to ask ourselves about this model of development is whether all who have developed in such a manner are always acting totally independently. Or, is it more likely that they often have someone behind the scenes—for example, a husband, a wife, a significant other or a secretary supporting them physically and emotionally? Such behind-the-scenes assistance could give the *impression* of independence, as in the phrase "behind every great man is a woman." Such an "ideal" model of development may not really be so ideal, since few can manage it; and even those who do so may have the tendency to become completely isolated. Such a model of development doesn't work; no one is completely independent. There are, however, degrees of both independence and dependence. We would be wise to rethink our expectations of the male model of development.

What about Women? Psychology, like medicine, has historically treated women like a lesser class of men.

In ancient Greece, no less a philosopher than Socrates said that "women are by no means inferior to men—all they need is a little more physical strength and energy of mind."[11]   For centuries, that attitude has been the best that women could expect to encounter.

Since the Middle Ages, Western society has seen women as a lesser version of men. Just as Eve was created from Adam's rib, Church doctrine held, so Woman should forever be subjugated to Man. Thomas Aquinas, the thirteenth century theologian, wrote that women were "defective by nature and 'misbegotten males.' "[12]

The early psychoanalysts held similar views; they cast women as weaker, imperfect versions of their ideal Independent Man. For decades, therefore, most psychological studies used only men as research subjects. And women, judged against this male standard, were often found lacking.

Dissatisfied with the male-based model of psychological development, some women *and* men have begun searching for a new model of the development of the self, one that considers the female psyche.

The New Female Model: The Interdependent Woman

Psychologists at the Stone Center for Developmental Services and Studies, at Wellesley College, have decided to take a fresh look at male development and how it might differ from female development. They have found that "Western culture sees power as coming from, and reflected by, independent action. The involvement of others implies individual weakness and lesser impact. . . . [A]utonomy, which usually means the capacity for independent action, is frequently and uncritically contrasted with connection. "[13]   Yet, as the Stone Center's Jean Baker Miller told *Time* magazine, "Women's sense of self and of worth is grounded in the ability to make and maintain relationships."[14]

"Can you do this independently, or can you only do it with others?" seems to be the critical question that men silently ask themselves.[15]   But, from a woman's point of view, the question could be restated as, "Can you do this with others, or can you only do it by yourself?"

"Relationship colors every aspect of a woman's life, according to the [Stone Center] researchers. Women use conversation to expand and understand relationships; men use talk to convey solutions, thereby ending conversation. Women tend to see people as mutually dependent; men view them as self-reliant. Women emphasize caring; men value freedom. Women consider actions within a context, linking one to the next; men tend to regard events as isolated and discrete."[16]

What about Men? Meanwhile, changing gender roles in our society, and evolving forms of socialization, are forcing a continued reconsideration of human development. One of the most surprising, yet far from irrational, results of this evolution is the push by many people—men and women—for a new *male* model of development.

GENDER AND POWER

> It is possible that power differences are in fact the major source of gender differences and difficulties between men and women.
>
> —*Judith Jordan,*
> *"The Movement of Mutuality and Power," 1991*

Many of the interpersonal challenges between men and women in our society derive from inequality rather than from any innate gender differences.

The Communication Gap

> Men mistakenly expect women to think, communicate, and react the way men do; women mistakenly expect men to feel, communicate, and respond the way women do. Becoming aware of the differences can dramatically reduce confusion when dealing with the opposite sex. When you remember that men are from Mars and women are from Venus, everything can be explained.
>
> —*John Gray,*
> *"Men Are from Mars, Women Are from Venus," 1992*

> If, like many men, one believes that human relations are fundamentally hierarchical, then playing on connection rather than status amounts to "pretending" there is no status—in other words, being deceptive. But those who tend to regard connection as the basic dynamic . . . see attempts to use status differences as manipulative and unfair.
>
> —*Deborah Tannen,*
> *"You Just Don't Understand: Women and Men in Conversation," 1990*

When they are not sure what to say, men are most apt to be silent, whereas women are more apt to express their uncertainty, or to reason out a position aloud. This can be interpreted as weakness on the part of women, or as obtuseness on the part of men, but it's really a matter of communication style.

Likewise, even among preschoolers, when they are attempting to influence the behavior of others, studies indicate that boys tend to take a more direct approach, whereas girls' efforts are far more indirect.[17] The indirectness typical of women and girls often is misunderstood as weakness or lack of power—especially if it is adopted by men or boys—and may, therefore, be taken advantage of. The directness favored by men and boys often is perceived as too abrupt, too pushy, or even rude—especially when it is adopted by women or girls, of whom it is not expected—and may, therefore, spur an angry response. Again, the problem is really a matter of communication style.

Men and women tend to differ not only in when they speak and what they say, but also in how they say it. This difference may be easier for us to see in another culture, such as that of Japan. Japanese is a tonal language—half spoken, half sung—in which the meaning of the words is very much dependent not only on the pronunciation of each syllable, or even on the stress it is given, but also on how high or low in tone it is spoken, compared with the rest of the word and sentence. Japanese children and Japanese women speak in the sing-songy way that conveys the most information the most easily. Japanese men, especially powerful Japanese men, may speak in a near monotone, leaving to their listeners the work of figuring out which words they meant to say. In ancient times, misinterpretation could be fatal. Today, it is merely a *faux pas*.

A similar pattern of expression is found in Western society.

It is telling that in the United States, as in Japan, the real "tough guys"— such as John Wayne, Clint Eastwood and Japan's Toshirô Mifune—have tended to speak in an inexpressive near monotone. It seems that those who have the most power have the least need to explain themselves—and that, by not explaining themselves, they demonstrate just how powerful they are.

On the other hand, in this tough-guy system, the lower-status members of society are likely to gain relationship skills that the upper crust lacks. "People with less power may need to be more aware of the feelings of those with more power so they can respond appropriately; in addition, leaders may be freer than followers about expressing their feelings. Thus, 'woman's intuition' may more accurately be referred to as 'subordinate's intuition.' "[18]

Relationship Styles

Male Relationships: The Quest for Power. Men, in Western society, seek power in relationships. Having been raised to value independence and strength, they are likely to devalue their relationships with others. They may see connection as representing dependence—that is, weakness, in the terms of the Independent Man—and perhaps a threat to their self-image. Aaron R. Kipnis expresses this attitude well, in his book *Knights Without Armor*: "I learned the codes for male conduct on the streets of Los Angeles and in the institutions of the juvenile justice system: be cool; never show fear, weakness, or pain; never back down from a fight; don't be a squealer; get your piece of the action any way you can."[19]

Our society has raised men to believe that they need to be able to do everything alone, to have all the answers—in other words, to be a rock. Male friends tend to leave much unspoken, dealing with emotion only obliquely. They tend not to offer sympathy—which would confirm a friend's weakness, and thus diminish his status—but rather to downplay one another's problems and suggest possible solutions. In essence, their ability to achieve intimacy is limited by their hierarchical framework, as if they must preserve the structure at any cost.

In truth, however, men have gotten a bad rap. They have been raised to be independent and to never cry or show emotion, and then, suddenly, have been expected to know how to be intimate and to show and share their emotions. This is not a reasonable expectation: The habits of a lifetime cannot be so easily overturned; the skills of emotional intimacy cannot be so easily learned. Such changes take time, and if they are to be widespread, require a number of motivating changes in the broader society.

Donald H. Bell, in his book *Being a Man*, describes men today as caught up "in the paradox of contemporary masculinity, suspended between the world in which they grew up and the one in which they must now live."[20]

Female Relationships: The Search for Connection. Women tend to seek connection in their relationships. Carol Gilligan notes that, whereas for men, identity takes precedence over intimacy, for women, intimacy goes along with identity. Women come to know themselves through their relationships with others. They may even define themselves by their relationships. As a result, a woman's level of attachment in a relationship tends to be greater than a man's.

According to Gilligan, women will use their sensitivity and their ability to hear other's voices to establish and maintain their relationships. And, women judge their ability to care for others critically, because of the high priority they assign to relationships. Women are raised to seek approval, which also plays a major role in these tendencies.

When Relationship Styles Collide. Men in our society are likely to be concerned about whether someone is trying to be one-up or one-down in a relationship, whereas women are likely to be more concerned about whether someone is attempting to get closer or pull away. Men are more likely to be concerned with preserving their independence; women, with furthering their interdependence. Men may believe that to have a relationship, they must be worthy; women, that to be worthy, they must have a relationship.

To paraphrase Deborah Tannen's explanation, for men, who are raised to see relationships primarily in terms of hierarchy, focusing on connection rather than status appears fundamentally false; for women, who are raised to see connection as essential to relationships, using status differences seems manipulative and unjust.[21]

Clearly, such different approaches can cause many difficulties between men and women. For instance, a wife may despair that her husband must not love or respect her, because he refuses to depend on her, while the husband may be convinced that his wife must not love or respect him, because she fails to acknowledge his efforts to stand on his own two feet.

These differing approaches to relationships also lie behind many of the differences in behavior that men and women find so puzzling.

Consider Tannen's surprise at the complaints of a fellow writer, who has been asked to notify his editor of where he will be, if he does any traveling, while his book is in production. When she is in the same situation, Tannen writes, it makes her feel needed and wanted. But her friend's reaction is very different: He can't imagine *not* feeling that, by being ordered to report his whereabouts, he was being framed as both controlled and lesser in rank. The female writer (Tannen) saw reporting her comings and goings to another person as a normal and expected part of a relationship with an editor. In her eyes, the request gave her status—she was important, because she was needed. The male writer saw such reporting as an imposition—a threat to his power and independence.   In his eyes, the request diminished a writer's status because it constrained his freedom.[22]

Consider, also, the classic example of the lost driver. Why do men so often refuse to ask directions? Because, to them, the benefits of obtaining additional information are outweighed by the costs of admitting that they need it.

In the male, hierarchical model of relationships, asking questions can be seen as a sign of inadequacy or stupidity. If one were smart, the reasoning goes, then one wouldn't need to ask. Yet in the female, interconnected model of relationships, asking questions can be seen as a way of creating or strengthening connections with others. Likewise, in the male model, asking for help can be seen as a sign of weakness and dependence—an acknowledgement of the superior skills or resources of the one whose aid is requested. Yet in the female model, asking for help can be a way of gaining status, rather than losing it.

The result, not surprisingly, is that women in our society are more likely to ask for help. When traveling, they are more likely to ask directions; in conversation, they are more likely to ask questions.

Human Relationships. The old stereotypes of appropriate male and female behavior are undergoing a transformation. We are moving in the direction of more equality and fewer, less-rigid stereotypes. Such changes are making themselves felt in many of our relationships, including the doctor/patient relationship.

Leadership Styles

> I have a style of walking around and stroking people. . . . I try to compliment them in front of their peers and go up and hug them. . . . A woman can show the warmth that a man often can't.
>
> —*Sandra Kurtzig, founder and president,*
> *ASK Computer Systems, Mountain View, Calif.*

Male Leadership. From the cradle, boys are encouraged to be strong, to be independent, to stand on their own two feet, to "be a man." They are taught never to show weakness. In organized sports, in arm-wrestling contests and schoolyard battles, in games such as King of the Hill, they are taught the importance of winning. By the time that they reach grade school, most boys have learned that it is good to win and shameful to lose. They have learned that it is better to act brave and invincible than to show pain, or fear, or weakness. They have learned that it is better to lead than to follow.

It is no surprise then, that in many men's eyes, leadership has to do with hierarchy and status, with being one-up or one-down.

It is this jockeying for position and concern about status that lie at the heart of our society's Independent Man model of male leadership.

Those who are leaders tend to exhibit such qualities. When male leaders see women who are showing their ability to *connect*, they often misjudge them as demonstrating a lack of independence, which in the men's view is the same

as showing incompetence and insecurity.

From early childhood, as Deborah Tannen puts it, "Giving orders and getting others to follow them was the way certain boys got to be and stay leaders. A command, by definition, distinguishes the speaker from the addressee and frames him as having more power."[23]

But is getting others to follow your lead all there is to leadership? Tannen gives us one such model of "leadership" that was considered successful only by the person who used it:

> [A] salesman boasted to his colleagues that he was one of the most powerful members of the sales staff. When he spoke at meetings, he was rarely crossed. He was proud of this, attributing it to his high status. In fact, no one crossed him because he was well known to have a quick temper and a nasty tongue, and no one wanted to be on the receiving end of his outbursts. The effect of fear is sometimes indistinguishable from the effect of respect.[24]

Was this salesman really powerful? Well, he believed that he was. He also believed that he was respected, when actually he was only feared. He would have been dumbfounded had he ever learned what his colleagues really thought of him; under the circumstances, however, honest feedback was not likely to be forthcoming. Although it is not generally considered leadership, his style of fear-based and hierarchical behavior *can* give power to those who employ it—but it is not without its costs, both to them and to those around them.

Let's look at some generally accepted models of male leadership: Generals George Patton and Norman Schwarzkopf; Presidents Franklin D. Roosevelt and John F. Kennedy; former Chrysler Corp. chairman Lee Iaccoca . . . . They all have in common the ability to lead large groups of people and to appear to be comfortable doing so. They all present an image of strength and dedication. They all are able to keep a cool head; able to make difficult decisions alone; and able to get others to take note of what they say.

Female Leadership. The style exhibited by women who have risen to positions of leadership in our society is somewhat different. It focuses on building teams, rather than on star players. It is often seen as a new style—less rigid and hierarchical, and more open and inclusive—distinct from the traditional management style of men. Sally Helgesen, author of *The Female Advantage: Women's Ways of Leadership*, describes this feminine style of management as involving more frank communication with employees, sharing information with them rather than withholding it, and leaving the office door open whenever possible. Juanita Kreps, a former U.S. Secretary of Commerce and a board member of several Fortune 500 companies, says "Women bring a problem-solving attitude that embraces coordination more than the masculine drive to have power."

This new style did not arise in a vacuum. Some women, even those in positions of substantial authority, opt to "avoid the appearance of giving orders because they fear subordinates will resent taking orders from a woman (a commonly held and partly substantiated view)."[25] Consider the experience of female lawyers in the 1970s and early 1980s:

> Some employees of feminist [law] firms—secretaries and receptionists—came to their jobs with images of women as professionals which were different from their images of male professionals. One lawyer commented that her staff felt her office would be a nice place and they wouldn't have to work hard. They objected to the work pressures . . . and worked at a slower pace than was common in male firms.[26]

The behaviors our society expects of leaders, such as assertiveness and aggression, have long been considered positive traits in men but negative traits in women. Actions that would cause a man to be considered an energetic up-and-comer may cause a woman to be labeled with the "b-word" (famously described by House Speaker Newt Gingrich's mother as the one that "rhymes with witch") by men and women alike.

With their management styles, some women have turned this problem into a solution, building not upon the one-upsmanship of the male model but rather upon the consensus-building skills that have long been the provenance of women, as the less-powerful partners in our society.

Leadership is never without its price, especially for women. Successful women traditionally have found themselves isolated among male peers who do not consider them to be truly equal. Though that situation has changed markedly in the past few decades, many women retain a fear of success that is a legacy of the era when a strong-minded woman was a freak and pariah. Dealing rationally with that fear can become a tremendous challenge.

But the leveling of the playing field continues. For instance, the recent rise in women's sports—fueled in large part by Title IX of the Civil Rights Act—is giving a generation of young woman their initiation into a once-male domain, and to the sports lingo and leadership styles that have had so much influence on America's business and professional culture.

GENDER AND THE DOCTOR/PATIENT RELATIONSHIP

"We can speculate on what goes on in the doctor/patient relationship," write Debra L. Roter and Judith A. Hall, in their book *Doctors Talking With Patients/Patients Talking With Doctors*, "from a large body of research on male and female social behavior in general. This general literature usually finds women to be more empathic, more socially skilled, more equalizing of status differences, and more "immediate" in their nonverbal behavior—that is, they make more attentive and warmer use of smiles, gazes, distance and touch."[27]

There are many differences between men and women in our society. So far, we have looked at culture, language, socialization, and genetic factors, and at the roles they play in gender differences. Now, we are going to explore the effect of gender differences on the doctor/patient relationship.

The Effect of Doctor Gender

When 70,000 *Consumer Reports* subscribers were surveyed about doctors, the results revealed that men rated male and female doctors about equally, whereas women rated female doctors as better in terms of caring, communication, and thoroughness.[28] A 1997 study of pediatric office visits found that children "were more satisfied with physicians of the same gender, while parents were more satisfied with female physicians."[29] Other studies, before and since, generally have found that patients who prefer doctors of a specific gender overwhelmingly prefer women practitioners.

The main reason appears to be that female doctors tend to have a different communication style than male doctors. They are more likely to encourage their patients, or to reassure them. They ask more questions of their patients and work harder at drawing them out.[30] Oh, and one more thing: "I don't like to be interrupted," one patient explained to a CNN reporter in the spring of 1996. Asked whether she meant that male doctors were less likely to answer questions, she replied, "That's been my experience."[31]

In addition, partly as a result of this different communication style, female doctors often are perceived as more caring and approachable—characteristics that many people look for in a doctor. Male and female doctors spend similar amounts of time talking about illness management, but female doctors also spend time on "social exchange," that is, on the kind of small talk that helps to create a friendly connection.[32]

Another possible explanation for the preference for female practitioners is the emphasis patients now place on prevention. A study at Saint Louis University's Health Sciences Center examined the medical records of 2,000 patients. That study, completed in the spring of 1995, compared the prevention practices of male and female physicians. The researchers found that female physicians were significantly more likely than their male counterparts to use widely recommended health screening tests: Patients of female physicians were fifty-six percent more likely to be given a cholesterol test, and fourty-seven percent more likely to be screened for cervical cancer. "Certain physicians need to focus more on prevention," concluded study author Matthew Kreuter, Ph.D.

The current preference for female doctors is particularly interesting given that, just a few decades ago, "lady doctors" were looked down upon by their patients, their nurses and their colleagues. Their skill, their knowledge, their authority, their commitment to their careers, and their femininity all were called into question. Female doctors were not and are not able to operate from the same position of power and strength as their male colleagues; but, as it happens, patients appear to prefer doctors who practice from a less-powerful position.

That is not to say that patients most prefer the doctors who are most feminine and least powerful. The most popular doctors are those who have found a way to combine the socialization of women and the socialization of doctors, or the weaker position of women and the stronger position of doctors, into a professional persona that is moderately powerful, moderately approachable, and nearly androgenous.[33]

Let's take a closer look at some of the ways in which doctor gender appears to affect the doctor/patient relationship.

Time with Patients. Data from the National Ambulatory Medical Care Survey showed that patients' appointments with female physicians lasted approximately five minutes longer, on average, than appointments with male physicians. When a female patient was seen by a female physician, the visits lasted almost six minutes longer, on average, than a visit by a female patient to a male physician.[34] As for what happened in that extra time that female doctors were found to have spent with their patients—most was devoted to talk.[35]

Likewise, in a 1997 study of pediatric office visits, "Female physician visits were twenty-nine percent longer than those with male physicians."[36] Again, that extra time was spent on talk.

Encouraging Communication. The talk between female doctors and their patients has been described as more positive, featuring partnership building, the asking of pertinent questions and the exchange of information. In that pediatric study, for instance, "[F]emale physicians engaged in more social exchange, more encouragement and reassurance . . . and more information gathering."[37]

When their patients are talking, female doctors are more likely to encourage them to continue. They use more "encouragers"—phrases like "yes," or "uh-huh," or "I see"—thereby encouraging their patients to continue. Women also engage in more psychosocial talk with their patients. They get their patients to converse about their lives in general.[38]

Not surprisingly, patients talk more with female doctors, and tend to feel more comfortable with them, than with their male counterparts.[39]

Discouraging Communication. Male doctors have been found to use more "discouragers"—techniques that helped to cut short their conversations with patients and allowed the doctors to maintain control. The men are more apt to fidget while a patient is talking; to consult a watch; to interrupt the patient; and to ask closed-ended questions, such as "Where does it hurt?," instead of open-ended questions, such as "Tell me where the pain is."[40]

Doctors of either gender have been found to be more likely to use a bored tone of voice when speaking with female patients.[41] This may indicate that physicians feel less of a need to compete with or to dominate a female patient than they feel when treating a male patient.

Changing the Subject. Patients often complain that doctors change the subject before anything has been settled. Female doctors have been found to be five times more likely to wait until they have reached agreement with the patient before changing the subject.[42]

Terms of Address. Perhaps because patients feel more comfortable with them than with their male counterparts, female doctors are more likely to be addressed by their first name by patients, and to be interrupted. Offsetting the slight annoyance of this potential loss of control, however, are substantial gains—in improved communication, improved care, and increased patient loyalty.

Nonverbal Communication. Doctors vary greatly in their ability to decode the nonverbal messages of their patients. In general, women are more skilled than men at interpreting such body language. Women also tend to be more aware of their *own* nonverbal communication, and in better control of it.

These capabilities have further implications that should be mentioned: Because they are more likely to be aware of their patients and their own unspoken signals, female doctors may be better able to avoid potential difficulties. Aiding in this regard is the greater effort female doctors generally exert to obtain patient agreement, a gap that is only broadened by the gender difference in nonverbal communication skills.

Doctors possessing these skills—so far, mostly female doctors—are more apt to be aware of a patient's unspoken doubts or questions. They are more able to elicit additional information that may be vital to the patient's care, and more apt to notice and deal with, at a pre-lawsuit stage, any unspoken reservations on the part of the patient.

It should be noted, of course, that some men do possess good verbal and nonverbal communication skills, and some women lack them. These abilities do not appear to be an inherent quality of women, but rather a result of lifelong socialization. Clearly, having been acquired, these abilities are acquirable. Like any other skills, these can be learned. The most effective way to do so is by attending communications workshops that stress role-playing and other active participation. A firmer grasp on the basics of nonverbal communication, as well as better verbal communication skills, is something that would benefit all doctors.

Caring. As Howard Brody, M.D., writes in *The Healer's Power*, "The cemetery is filled not with the corpses of patients who died because their overinvolved physicians became irrational and ineffective, but rather with those of sufferers whose physicians attended to their diseases but failed to heal because of the multiple characterological barriers that cause *physicians* not to get close enough."[43]

In their professional training, doctors are taught to not get too close to their patients, for fear that they might lose their objectivity and thereby become ineffective. But patients generally do not suffer because their doctors care too much. It may be a lack of caring on the part of their physician that causes them to suffer instead. It is the "care" part of health care that has been left out. And it is this element that needs to be reintroduced.

Empathy—that is, understanding and feeling what it is like to be a patient—is a skill that had been ignored by the health-care establishment for much of the last century. But as patients have begun to express more and more dissatisfaction with the care they receive, the industry has taken note. Some doctors now are being trained to empathize with their patients by being subjected to the experiences of a patient. Thus, they learn what it is like to place themselves in others' hands.

The February 1995 issue of *Consumer Reports* describes one such program:

''When new resident physicians in family medicine report to work at the Long Beach Memorial Medical Center in Long Beach, Calif., they're assigned to a hospital bed, hooked up to an intravenous line, and subjected to various tests and exams. The reason, oddly enough, is that they're young and healthy.''[44]

It is for good reason that similar programs now exist in many schools and hospitals, including Harvard Medical School, Michigan State University and Rhode Island Hospital. Students and practitioners at these institutions are being trained in communication and listening skills not only because it is good medicine, but also because it is good self-defense: Many doctors who have been sued for malpractice say they believe no suit would have been filed had they had a better relationship with their patients. And patients who file lawsuits against their doctors cite communication issues in more than 70 percent of their malpractice complaints.[45]

Empathic and relational skills—both physical and emotional—have been a part of the socialization of women for centuries. Female physicians, therefore, are likely to bring these skills into the doctor/patient relationship. Men, on the other hand, have been socialized to be independent, self-controlled, and task-oriented. The energies of male physicians, as a result, tend to be mostly directed at the physical aspect of caring.

But the costs of ignoring a patient's emotional needs may be tremendous. A doctor may fail to determine a patient's treatment objectives, or may miss important diagnostic information. Healing may be seriously impaired if a doctor does not deal with a patient's mental as well as physical condition.

Modern medicine has rediscovered the critical role of the mind-body connection, and its effect on the immune system and on the speed of healing. This can be seen in the placebo effect, in which patients convinced that they are receiving an effective treatment recover as if they were, and in what some researchers call the ''nocebo'' effect, in which people convinced that they are receiving a treatment with adverse effects exhibit those effects. For instance, in a study of an experimental chemotherapy agent, cancer patients were divided into two groups: one got the drug, the other, an inert substance. ''One-third of the placebo group experienced hair loss—simply because they *believed* they would. Roughly the same proportion of the chemotherapy group experienced hair loss.''[46]

It is when patients are cared for emotionally as well as physically, when healing bonds are forged between doctor and patient, that healing is most likely to take place.

Thoroughness. ''Mostly, male and female doctors did not differ [in thoroughness or technical expertise]. However, female doctors scored much higher on the frequency with which they checked for breast and cervical cancer in women. When dealing with medical tasks uniquely relevant to their own sex, these women may have experienced a heightened identification of empathy that led them to be more thorough.''[47] That was one of the conclusions drawn in a study that focused its attention on the technical expertise of male and female doctors at 16 ambulatory care practices in the Boston area.[48]

Overall, however, no appreciable differences in thoroughness were found. Male and female doctors were equally competent.

The Effect of Patient Gender

Thoroughness. Although doctor gender did not appear to influence thoroughness in the ambulatory care study cited above, patient gender did. Ear infections were treated more aggressively in boys than in girls; urinary tract infections were treated more aggressively in girls than in boys. "It appears, then, that doctors are likely to follow accepted procedure best when treating the sex that is 'known' for the condition. . . . Of course this makes no rational sense. A girl with an ear infection will suffer the same complications and possible permanent damage as a boy if the condition is not treated properly."[49]

Physician Comfort and Efficacy. Whenever a doctor is dealing with a patient of a different age, gender, culture, or social class, communication has the potential to become a problem that requires special attention. But doctors have even more to be on guard against than one might think, when dealing with patients who differ from themselves.

In a study conducted by the American Association for the Advancement of Science, doctors were divided into two groups. Each member of both groups was given the same list of symptoms with a misleading piece of information. But doctors in one group also were given candy—as a thank-you, they were told —while doctors in the other group were given nothing. The doctors who had been given the candy were found to be more likely to diagnose the patient's problem correctly. The study concluded that when a doctor felt happy, he or she was far more likely to do a good job. It also concluded that healing a patient was seen by the doctors as more valuable than a larger paycheck.[50]

A separate study of doctors found that male doctors were happier seeing male patients than female patients, and that doctors were happier seeing healthy patients than ones who were suffering.[51] This should come as no surprise since, in general, people are happiest dealing with people who are most like them; and since, in general, healthy people tend to be more cheerful and more pleasant to be with. It follows naturally, then, that doctors would most enjoy seeing healthy people who were much like themselves.

But, because most doctors are male and most patients are female, most doctors are likely to spend the greater part of their time with patients who are unlike them. (One study put the ratio of physician office visits by women to office visits by men at approximately 1.5 visits to 1.[52]) The disparity between doctors and patients is likely to become even wider when socioeconomic factors, as well as gender, are taken into account.

The association between physician happiness and the effectiveness of treatment decisions means that these conclusions about comfort levels, however obvious, have disturbing implications.

Communication. Women, in general, ask more questions in conversation than do men; they also are more likely to ask for help. It is not startling to learn that female patients do the same. As a result, they tend to receive more information from their doctors than do male patients. Another finding in studies on the effects of gender on doctor/patient communication is that physicians of either gender, when interacting with female patients, used a flatter, more "boring" tone of voice. The interactions of doctors with female patients were, in general, more low-key; doctors had less of an active and dominating manner with them.[53]

Frequency of Care. Women are more frequent users of health-care services than are men. Statistics on physician's visits in the United States show that from 1928 to 1974, the average woman had 5.6 doctor's visits per year, versus 4.3 visits per year for the average man. Hospital admissions for the same period also were much higher for female patients than for males.[54] Women received more medical care, had more return visits, were prescribed more drugs, and were given more tests than men.[55]

Some of this disparity, naturally, is attributable to gynecological and obstetrical visits. Another factor, often unacknowledged, is the greater willingness of women both to acknowledge weakness and to seek help. Women are, in general, more likely to make appointments for routine preventive care; more willing to seek help when they are unwell; and swifter to notice and acknowledge that they may be unwell. In fact, in Western society, women often are the gatekeepers for health care, making most of the medical decisions—and appointments—for their families.[56]

Yet, while the evidence shows that women visit doctors and hospitals more often than men, they are given more tests and more medication, and they return to their doctors more frequently, there also is the disturbing and somewhat incongruous data that they often receive less care.

For example, though women are given more tranquilizers than men, they also are given less pain medication than men who have the same conditions and the same amount of pain. They are given more tests, but most of those are routine. Women are not taken as seriously as men when they present with symptoms of potential heart ailments—nor does the problem end with diagnosis. Female heart patients tend to be given less aggressive treatment than men with the same condition—even though heart disease is the leading killer of both men and women.[57]

SUMMARY

What accounts for the differences, in practice style and patient care, between male and female doctors?

Perhaps the most important factor is the secondary role of women in our society, which gives female doctors, like women in general, a weaker but more approachable image. Our culture's socialization of women likewise is responsible for female doctors being more relationship-oriented and possessing stronger communication skills.

Ironically, the weaker doctor role that has been forced upon female practitioners turns out to be more effective both for treating patients and for pleasing them than the traditional posture of distant authority. We all can learn from this. Indeed, we must, for as our society becomes more equitable, the differences in men's and women's socialization are melting away.

Meanwhile, the key to minimizing the adverse effects of gender on the doctor/patient relationship lies in carefully sifting through what is real, what is personal, and what is culturally influenced. The first step is to gain a greater awareness of our own gender tendencies and biases. With such awareness, we will be far less likely to be caught in the web of gender discrimination.

NOTES

1. Tomson Highway, "It's Never O.K.: A Personal Viewpoint," plenary address presented at *It's Never O.K., The Third International Conference on Sexual Exploitation by Health Professionals, Psychotherapists and Clergy*, Toronto, Ontario, Canada, Oct. 15, 1994.

2. Bruce Handy, "Deconstructing Leo: What the Men Don't Get, the Teen Girls Understand," *Time*, March 20, 1998, 53.

3. Patricia Aburdene and John Naisbitt, *Megatrends for Women* (New York: Villard Books, 1992), 2.

4. Margaret Mead, *Sex and Temperament in Three Primitive Societies* (New York: William Morrow and Company, 1935), 56, 213.

The Tchambuli people whom Mead studied in Samoa are only one of several known societies in which female aggression is the norm. Another is described by Victoria Katherine Burbank in *Fighting Women: Anger and Aggression in Aboriginal Australia* (Berkeley: University of California Press, 1994).

5. Lionel Tiger, *Men in Groups* (New York: Random House, 1969), 44.

6. The phrase "the naked ape," like the field of evolutionary biology, was popularized by Desmond Morris, in his book *The Naked Ape: A Zoologist's Study of the Human Animal* (New York: McGraw-Hill, 1967).

7. Sigmund Freud used this phrase in his 1912 work *On the Universal Tendency to Debasement in the Sphere of Love*, Section III.

8. Barbara Rudolph, "Why Can't a Woman Manage More Like . . . a Woman?" *Time*, Special Issue, Women: The Road Ahead. 136 (1990), 53.

9. The Sphinx of Grecian mythology, a semi-divine creature, perched high on a rock outside of Thebes and asked the same riddle of each passer-by: "What is it that goes on four feet in the morning, two feet at midday, and three in the evening, and has but a single voice." One person after another, unable to find the correct answer, forfeited his or her life to the Sphinx. Then came Oedipus, who correctly answered: "Man," because people crawl in their infancy, walk in their middle years, and in their old age, may hobble upon a cane. On hearing his answer, the Sphinx hurled herself to her death—immediately making Thebes a much more popular travel destination.

10. Gail Sheehy, *New Passages: Mapping Your Life Across Time* (New York: Random House, 1995), 148.

11. Reay Tannahill, *Sex In History* (Chelsea, Miss.: Scarborough House, 1992), 93.

12. Aburdene and Naisbitt, *Megatrends for Women*, 114.

13. Alexandra G. Kaplan, "Dichotomous Thought and Relational Processes in Therapy," Work in Progress No. 35 (Wellesley, Mass.: The Stone Center for Developmental Services and Studies, Wellesley College, 1988), 9.

14. Jean Baker Miller's comments are reported in an article by Anastasia Toufexis, "Coming from a Different Place: Men and Women Just Don't See Things the Same Way. Some Surprising New Studies of Schoolgirls Show Why," *Time,* Special Issue, Women: The Road Ahead, 136 (1990), 64-65.

15. Kaplan, "Dichotomous Thought and Relational Processes in Therapy," 9.

16. Anastasia Toufexis, "Coming from a Different Place: Men and Women Just Don't See Things the Same Way. Some Surprising New Studies of Schoolgirls Show Why," *Time,* Special Issue, Women: The Road Ahead, 136 (1990), 65.

17. Judith V. Jordan, "The Movement of Mutuality and Power," Work in Progress No. 53 (Wellesley, Mass.: The Stone Center for Developmental Services and Studies, Wellesley College, 1991), 3.

18. Diane E. Papalia and Sally Wendkos Olds, *Psychology*, 2nd ed. (New York: McGraw-Hill Book Company, 1985), 426.

19. Aaron R. Kipnis, *Knights Without Armor: A Practical Guide for Men in the Quest of Masculine Soul* (Los Angeles, Calif.: St. Martin's Press, 1991), 165.

20. Donald H. Bell, *Being a Man: The Paradox of Masculinity* (Lexington, Mass.: The Lewis Publishing Company, 1982), 35.

21. Deborah Tannen, *You Just Don't Understand: Women and Men in Conversation* (New York: Ballantine Books, 1990), 38.

22. Tannen, *You Just Don't Understand*, 39.

23. Tannen, *You Just Don't Understand*, 39.

24. Tannen, *You Just Don't Understand*, 182.

25. Cynthia Fuchs Epstein, *Women in Law* (Garden City, N.Y: Anchor Press/Doubleday, 1983), 157.

26. Fuchs Epstein, *Women in Law*, 156-157.

27. Debra L. Roter and Judith A. Hall, *Doctors Talking with Patients/Patients Talking with Doctors: Improving Communication in Medical Visits* (Westport, Conn.: Auburn House, 1992), 62.

28. "How Is Your Doctor Treating You?" *Consumer Reports*, 60 (February 1995), 81.

29. Jane Bernzweig, John I. Takayama, Ciaran Phibbs, Catherine Lewis, and Robert H. Pantell, "Gender Differences in Physician-Patient Communication: Evidence from Pediatric Visits," *Archives of Pediatrics & Adolescent Medicine*, 151 (June 1997): 586-591.

30. Bernzweig, Takayama, Phibbs, Lewis, and Pantell, "Gender Differences in Physician-Patient Communication," 586-591.

31. It is an experience confirmed in numerous studies of doctor/patient communication.

32. Bernzweig, Takayama, Phibbs, Lewis, and Pantell, "Gender Differences in Physician-Patient Communication," 586-591.

33. P.R. Yarnold, *et al.*, "Androgeny Predicts Empathy for Trainees in

Medicine," *Perceptual Motor Skills*, 77 (October 1993), 576-578.

34. Roter and Hall, *Doctors Talking with Patients*, 62.

35. Roter and Hall, *Doctors Talking with Patients*, 63.

36. Bernzweig, Takayama, Phibbs, Lewis, and Pantell, "Gender Differences in Physician-Patient Communication," 586-591.

37. Bernzweig, Takayama, Phibbs, Lewis, and Pantell, "Gender Differences in Physician-Patient Communication," 586-591.

38. Roter and Hall, *Doctors Talking with Patients*, 44.

39. Roter and Hall, *Doctors Talking with Patients*, 64.

40. Roter and Hall, *Doctors Talking with Patients*, p. 44.

41. Roter and Hall, *Doctors Talking with Patients*, p. 45.

42. Deborah Tannen, *Talking from 9 to 5: How Women's and Men's Conversational Styles Affect Who Gets Heard, Who Gets Credit, and What Gets Done at Work* (New York: William Morrow and Company, 1994), p. 172.

43. Dr. Howard Brody, *The Healer's Power* (New Haven, Conn.: Yale University Press, 1992), p. 264.

44. "Changing Medical Education: Let's Play Patient," *Consumer Reports*, 60 (February 1995), p. 83.

45. "Changing Medical Education," *Consumer Reports*, p. 83.

46. Larry Dossey, "Medical Hexing: The Nocebo Effect and You," *Bottom Line/Health*, June 1998, 15.

47. Roter and Hall, *Doctors Talking with Patients*, p. 123.

48. Those interested in learning more about this study may wish to consult the study report, by Judith A. Hall, R.H. Palmer, E.J. Orav, J.L. Hargraves, E.A. Wright and A.T. Louis, "Performance, Quality, Gender and Professional Role: A Study of Physicians and Nonphysicians in Sixteen Ambulatory Care Practices," *Medical Care*, 28 (1990), 489-501.

49. Roter and Hall, *Doctors Talking with Patients*, p. 123.

50. "The Happier the Doctor, the Better the Diagnosis, Study Finds," *The Providence Journal-Bulletin*, Feb. 23, 1995, p. A-4.

51. Roter and Hall, *Doctors Talking with Patients*, p. 43.

52. Roter and Hall, *Doctors Talking with Patients*, p. 43.

53. Roter and Hall, *Doctors Talking with Patients*, p. 45.

54. Andrew C. Twaddle, *A Sociology of Health* (Saint Louis: Mosby, 1977), p. 152.

55. Roter and Hall, *Doctors Talking with Patients*, p. 53.

56. Consider, for example, the cough-syrup commercials for Robitussin, which proudly declare that the company's products are "recommended by 'Doctor Mom.' "

57. Aburdene and Naisbitt, *Megatrends for Women*, p. 135.

— 2 —

Sexuality

SEXUALITY: 1. the state or quality of being sexual; 2. a. interest in or concern with sex; b. sexual drive or activity

Webster's New World Dictionary,
Third College Edition, 1994

What is sex—and how does it differ from sexuality? One definition of sex has to do with the differences between males and females, but the term today is more commonly used to indicate sexual relations, or being involved in a sexual manner: going to bed, sleeping together, having sex, sexual intercourse, making love, doing the wild thing. For the sake of clarity, this book embraces the latter meaning of "sex," using it to indicate sexual intercourse or other sexual acts. In this usage, "sex" can become an adjective; for example, one may "feel sexy" or be a "sexy woman or man"; one has sexual fantasies or sexual organs. "Sex" can also be used as a noun, as in "they had sex."

The field that studies humans and sex currently uses the term "sexuality," because it is a more holistic concept. It encompasses feelings about ourselves and others as sexual beings, including attractiveness and body image; ideas and experiences about relationships; and a healthy concept of choice, responsibility, and mutual interaction. The Sexuality Information and Education Council of the United States (SIECUS) offers this working definition: "Sexuality encompasses not only anatomy and biochemistry (what most people have come to think of as 'sex'), but also gender roles, personality, thoughts, feelings and behaviors. The term 'sexuality' refers to who people are as men and women, and not to body parts, reproduction, or physical acts."

Sexuality is a basic physical and emotional facet of human life. In her book *Women's Wisdom, Women's Bodies*, Dr. Christiane Northrup writes that "Our culture associates sexuality with genitalia, even though the expression of sexuality involves much more than that. Humans are the only primates whose sexual desire and functioning are not necessarily related to the reproductive cycle.''[1]

We all know that men and women are taught to think differently about sex and sexuality. Men more often think of the act of sexual intercourse, whereas women more often think of the larger relationship. The concept that men tend to emphasize would be defined as sex; the concept that women tend to emphasize would be defined more as sexuality. And herein lies one of the biggest differences not only between sex and sexuality, but also between men and women: in how we think of sex.

SEXUALITY IN WESTERN CULTURE

Heterosexuality

We all know the sexual stereotypes: men are the seducers, and women the seduced. This statement highlights the traditional Western approach to sexuality: the dominant role of males, and the submissive role of females. A further stereotype is that men are powerful but are victims of their own sexuality, whereas women are masters of their own sexuality but are victims of everything else. These categorical views are a direct result of the notion of sex as power, a reflection of the darker side of our sexual culture. These are views of beastly men and predatory women. But how are these images created and sustained?

In their book *Mystery Dance on the Evolution of Human Sexuality*, authors Lynn Margulis and Ann Dorion Sagan attribute the problem to the rigidity of our society's current childrearing structures. "Part of the problem with the relationship between the sexes later in life stems from the fact that we are, most of us, not only born of but reared by women," the authors write. "The central figure in the infantile life of both boys and girls is female—a mother who is loved and hated, who provides and denies, who coddles and neglects."[2]

Northrup, on the other hand, traces the problem to a socialization that drives women to preserve relationships—at any cost. "Women have been socialized for centuries to put their physical bodies at risk in order to sustain interpersonal relationships that really don't support them or their well-being."[3]

It is probable that both factors play a part. But surely, our society's image of heterosexuality must hinge upon the behavior of both men and women. Donald Bell, in his book *Being a Man*, offers this straightforward, first-person account of adolescent socialization:

> As we grew up, it was clear that as boys we learned different lessons about sexuality and love than those learned by our girlfriends. For boys, sex often seemed an end in itself and a means to succeed in a competitive masculine world. . . . [W]e either "scored" or "failed." Our guideline for behavior never was to become emotionally committed. We tried to get as much as we could while giving as little of ourselves as possible . . . . to be a member, as we said, of the "Four F" club: find 'em, feel 'em,

fuck 'em and forget 'em.

For girls, however, sexuality was expressed less directly and was often used as an emblem of one's feminine attractiveness . . . . According to the rules of the game, girls who valued themselves needed to avoid sexual encounters as much as possible and concentrate their main efforts on having and keeping boyfriends. From this, in turn, stemmed our own underlying disrespect for those girls whom we actually persuaded to "put out."[4]

Likewise, Michael S. Kimmel, in his essay for the book *Transforming a Rape Culture*, writes that "Women have been assigned the role of asexual gatekeeper; women decide, metaphorically and literally, who enters the desired garden of earthly delights, and who doesn't. . . . A man's job is to wear down her resistance."[5]

Other Sexualities

> If homosexuality were the normal way, God would have made Adam and Bruce.
>
> —*Anita Bryant,*
> *1977*

> It doesn't matter what you do in the bedroom, as long as you don't do it in the street and frighten the horses.
>
> —*Beatrice Stella Campbell,*
> *circa 1905*

Homosexuality. The evidence is overwhelming that homosexuality is an integral part of nature. In most of the species with two genders that humans have bothered to study, homosexuality has been observed. There is increasing scientific support for a genetic and biochemical basis for homosexuality.[6] What is more, despite the role that environment is thought to play, even the strongest of societal pressures have notably failed to significantly affect rates of homosexuality in a human population.[7]

Within some societies, the majority of young people engage in same-gender sex before marriage. In other societies, same-gender sex is regarded as an abomination and is discouraged by stiff social or criminal penalties. But in all cultures that have been studied, the incidence of adult homosexuality appears to be approximately the same. And in the United States, the incidence of adult homosexuality has not increased over the years, despite increasing acceptance of nonheterosexual relationships.[8]

Though homosexuals have long been the target of abuse and stereotyping, the reality is that they are little different from their neighbors. Some are assertive, some are meek. Some are bookish, some are flamboyant. Some are liberal, some are conservative. "Large-scale studies have found that homosexual men act in most ways like heterosexual men and that lesbians (homosexual women) are very similar to heterosexual women. The major difference is in the sex of the person preferred as a partner."[9]

Bisexuality. People who "swing both ways" may be shunned by the heterosexual and homosexual populations alike. Both segments of society may consider them to be traitors to their gender and sexual roles.

Yet psychologists describe human sexuality, like the human psyche, as comprising a balance of "male" and "female" traits. Sigmund Freud, the father of psychoanalysis, viewed humankind as universally disposed toward bisexuality. It was his belief that everyone has male and female "sides," each of which is attracted to its opposite gender, but that most people repress one of the two sides. For Freud, it was the idea of exclusive heterosexuality that presented a problem.

"Mostly, though, we'd rather not think about bisexuality. . . . [It] has been written out of our literature: early publishers simply rewrote the genders of male love objects in Plato's 'Symposium' and some of Shakespeare's sonnets; more often, schools just teach around them. Bisexuality even disappears from many sex surveys, which count people with any same-sex behavior as homosexual."[10]

Not only is bisexuality seen as a challenge to the notion of monogamy—due largely to the mistaken belief that being bisexual necessitates involvement with more than one person—but also, it wreaks havoc with accepted gender roles. Although a gay man can be considered to play the role of a woman, and a lesbian woman can be considered to play the role of a man, a bisexual man or woman does not fit neatly into either pigeonhole. Our divided, yes-or-no culture cannot cope with anything it cannot readily categorize; it can find no place for people who insist on playing both gender roles, or neither. Dr. Stanley M. Aronson, in an essay that appeared in *The Providence Journal-Bulletin*, expressed this problem well: "Society, with its laws and customs, has little tolerance for ambiguity; it insists that each citizen be of one sex or the other, much like the rigidity demanded in a two-party political system."[11]

It is particularly ironic, therefore, that many of our cultural icons—and many of this century's sexual icons, including Billie Holliday, Marlene Dietrich, Cary Grant, James Dean and, more recently, Madonna—are believed to have enjoyed sexual relationships with both men and women.[12]

Implications for the Doctor/Patient Relationship

Estimates of the percentage of the population that is homosexual vary, in part because varying definitions of homosexuality have been used. But taking the most-cited estimates of roughly five percent to ten percent, we can calculate that about one in every ten to twenty adults is homosexual—or bisexual, since, as was noted above, the two categories are often combined. The representation of homosexuals in the patient population is likely to be higher, not only because homosexual relationships are less likely to result in children, and therefore are likely to leave their participants with more disposable income, but also because gays and lesbians may, for a number of reasons, be more health-conscious than the general population.[13] We know, therefore, that every doctor is likely to see a significant number of patients who are nonheterosexual. So every doctor needs to be prepared to treat these patients effectively and respectfully, and to deal with their concerns—which, for the most part, are the same as any patient's.

THE STUDY OF SEX AND SEXUALITY

Until the 1940s, sexuality was considered literally unspeakable and was practically ignored. That is when Alfred Kinsey began his groundbreaking research. He surveyed people about what they did, sexually, and even made some observations of people engaged in sexual intercourse. He was followed, in the 1950s, by William H. Masters and Virginia E. Johnson, and their Reproductive Biology Foundation. They went on to analyze what happens in the human body during sexual excitement and intercourse. While the methods and conclusions of these pioneers have been faulted, their work and subsequent studies have helped to shed light on the reasons for sexual dysfunction, as well as on what constitutes normal sexual function and practices.

There are several reasons, however, why human sexuality continues to resist scientific inquiry:

1.　The subject is still often viewed as embarrassing.
2.　The sexual part of ourselves is too familiar and automatic; it is something we are accustomed to dealing with only on emotional, subconscious level. It can be difficult for us to elevate the subject to a rational, conscious level.
3.　The analysis of sex and sexuality is simply not a part of the Western tradition.

Eastern cultures have been much more successful in making sexuality something integral to, rather than something divorced from, the larger society. The *Kama Sutra* and the Japanese and Chinese "pillow books" are written, and viewed, not as pornography but as literature, or art, or straightforward how-to manuals, or some combination of the three. There is even a tradition of sacred sexuality, as is evinced in Tantric yoga and other Eastern disciplines.

But over the past few centuries, Western culture has increasingly come to view sexuality as not fit for polite society. It has repressed the study, analysis, and rational consideration of the topic. Sexuality has been restricted to the bedroom, to pornography, and, of course, to commercialism.

CULTURAL MYTHS AND MESSAGES

Just as repression is unhealthy for an individual, it also is unhealthy for a society. And our society is in recovery from centuries of repression. We need to unload some of the baggage that has accumulated along the way, and rethink some of the messages that our culture has been transmitting.

The Myth of Entitlement

Among the maladjusted cultural messages we need to reassess is the myth of male sexual entitlement. For centuries, young men in our culture have grown up believing that any woman who somehow inspires their lust is obligated to do something about it. And if this woman has gone so far as to accept a movie or dinner or some other commodity, then they consider her to have been bought and paid for. "She owes me," some might say. This is certainly one of the oldest and most persistent adolescent myths.

Not surprisingly, it has been discovered that the encouragement or even the tacit acceptance of this attitude can contribute to the more overtly violating behaviors such as harassment, abuse and rape.

The "Need" for Release

Then there is the myth that it is dangerous or harmful for a male *not* to immediately relieve his sexual tension. The real risk is from the myth itself, which is especially dangerous when combined with the myth of entitlement.

This attitude has been another major contributor to the phenomenon of date rape, as well as rape in general, and to the abuse of clients by physical and mental health practitioners.

The Fast-Food Culture

Both of these viewpoints seem to be reinforced in our culture by the prevalence of nonsexual messages that encourage people to take what they want, when they want it. Consider this sampling of recent advertising slogans:

McDonald's:	"You deserve a break today"
Burger King:	"Have it your way"
Pop Secret microwave popcorn:	"Instant, total gratification"
Diet Coke:	"Right now!"
Sprite:	"Obey your thirst"
Nike:	"Just do it"

The Sexual Scoreboard

"In locker rooms and on playgrounds across the country, men are taught that the goal of every encounter with women is to score. Men are supposed to be ever ready for sex, constantly seeking sex, and constantly seeking to escalate every encounter so that intercourse will result."[14]

The Myth of the Helpless Male

Men in our society may believe they can't help themselves. They may even be honored by their peers for having sexual urges so strong that they cannot control them. It is only among men in positions of power, however, that this ''uncontrollable'' sexuality is seen as admirable.

Traditionally, a high-status man who ''just couldn't help himself'' with a maid or a ''loose woman'' or a girl from the wrong side of the tracks—or with a groupie or a secretary or a congressional aide—would be subject only to a little good-natured joshing. A poor kid from a bad neighborhood who ''just couldn't help himself'' with someone of even lower social status than himself also would be likely to suffer no legal or social sanctions. But what if this bad boy's victim turned out to be a local debutante, or the police chief's daughter?

THE ISSUE OF POWER

Whenever sex becomes a tool to control, to demean, or to injure, it becomes a serious threat. This is the dark side of sexuality. And in Western society, sex, love, and dominance are dangerously confused.

Domination and Desire

Power is viewed as sexy in men, and submission or capitulation as sexy in women; thus, men learn that it is advantageous to exert power over others. This image may help to explain our society's high rate of rape and other sex-linked crimes, as rape is primarily an act of domination with intent to injure. It is a short step from the belief that power is sexy in men to the belief that it is sexy for men to exert power over others, with or without their consent.

Athletic Aggression and Military Macho

When aggression is regarded as a mark of virility, any limit that is placed on that virility can be seen as a threat to the very ability to be aggressive. This tangled belief appears to lie at the root of our society's tolerance of sexual transgressions by athletes and soldiers, of whom aggression is demanded.

The publicity accorded to boxer Michael Tyson's rape of Miss America contender Desiree Washington ''underscores our particular fascination with athletes, and the causal equation we make between athletes and sexual aggression. From [incidents involving] athletic teams and individual players at campuses across the nation, we're getting the message that our young male athletes, trained for fearless aggression on the field, are translating that into a predatory sexual aggression in relationships with women. Columnist Robert Lipsyte calls it 'the varsity syndrome—winner take all, winning at any cost, violence as a tool, aggression as a mark of masculinity.' ''[15]

A similar response was seen to Navy's Tailhook scandal, in which top aviators at a convention allegedly lined the halls of their hotel to denigrate and grope female passers-by. And to the more recent Army scandal, in which career soldiers came forward at substantial risk to themselves to accuse a higher-ranking official of sexual harassment. These and other high-profile embarassments have forced the U.S. armed forces to begin confronting problems in their own ranks, problems that formerly were dismissed with a boys-will-be-boys kind of attitude.

Though others may see the sexual excesses of some American athletes and military men as separate issues, Michael S. Kimmel groups these phenomenon under a single heading, which he calls the problem of men in groups.

"Men's fear of being judged a failure as a man in the eyes of other men leads to a certain homosocial element within the heterosexual encounter: men often will use their sexual conquest as a form of currency to gain status among other men. Such homosocial competition contributes to the strange hearing impairment that men experience in any sexual encounter, a socialized deafness that leads us to hear 'no' as 'yes' . . . to always go for it, to score."[16]

SEXUALITY IN OTHER CULTURES

Our culture's ideas and attitudes about sexuality are not universal; not all cultures think about sex in the same way. Eastern cultures have a view of sexuality that is much more positive and much less separate from other aspects of life. In some cultures, sexuality is valued as an art form and even has religious aspects. For instance, in Tantric yoga—one part of a tradition that sees sexuality as an integral part of spirituality—the "giver" is seen as equal to the "receiver." Western civilizations have much to learn in this regard.

That is not to say, however, that Eastern cultures have eliminated all sexual concerns. The ancient physician Sun Szu-mo is said to have opined that it would be wonderful if the mind could always be "serene and entirely untroubled by thoughts of sex. . . . But among 10,000 men there is perhaps one who can achieve this."[17] Some things apparently have changed little since his time.

SEXUALITY IN THE DOCTOR/PATIENT RELATIONSHIP

All health-care professionals are challenged by their sexuality and the sexuality of their patients on a daily basis. Not all practitioners are aware of this challenge on a conscious level. Yet awareness of one's own sexuality and that of one's patients, and of the interaction between the two, is critical to providing a safe and healing environment. We who play the role of doctor have both a responsibility and an opportunity to integrate the many aspects of ourselves.

"Where there is no fact, fantasy and fallacy flourish."[18] The key to safely dealing with sexuality and the doctor/patient relationship is to become aware of the facts—personal, as well as general.

Some facts about sexuality have been presented above, but information of a personal nature must be gathered by the individual practitioner, through personal assessment of ideas and behaviors.

First, it is necessary to consider and to monitor the practitioner's own sexuality. Among the questions to consider: What is your sexual makeup? Your orientation? What and how strong are your sexual needs and wants? Are they being met? How do you look upon patients? As potential partners? As people to flirt with? In other words, what sexual agenda does the physician bring to the doctor/patient relationship? Some of this information about yourself, you may already know. Some of it, you may need to explore further. Guidelines for making such an assessment can be found in Part III of this book, the Patient Protection Protocol.

Second, it is important to consider the patient's sexuality. With most patients, it is important to stay attuned to the signals that the patient is sending. With practice, this can become second nature. Asking oneself questions like these can be helpful: What is this particular patient's sexual makeup? What is his or her sexual agenda? How does he or she perceive me sexually? As a potential partner? As someone to flirt with and get attention from? As someone to seduce? As sexually irrelevant? This information may not be readily apparent, but being aware of any signals that are present can be very helpful. You may already be picking up more signals than you realize. For instance, you may feel nervous or uneasy about certain patients without being sure why.

Becoming more aware of your own sexuality and your own sexual agenda will make it easier to filter out your own reactions, so that you can focus on the patient's verbal and nonverbal cues. When these personal and professional assessments have been made, the doctor is better prepared to care for patients. It is important to remember, however, that the doctor is always responsible for maintaining professional boundaries—that is, for keeping all interaction on a purely professional level—regardless of the patient's attitudes or behaviors.

How can doctors prepare to care for patients in the best and most appropriate manner? We need to consider ourselves and others as sexual subjects, rather than as sexual objects; as masters of our own destiny, rather than victims of our own sexuality; as people, rather than as things. With a change in perspective like this, we will begin to see ourselves and others differently.

NOTES

1. Christiane Northrup, *Women's Wisdom, Women's Bodies: Creating Physical and Emotional Health and Healing* (New York: Bantam Books, 1995), 225.

2. Lynn Margulis and Ann Dorion Sagan, *Mystery Dance on the Evolution of Human Sexuality* (New York: Summit Books, 1991), 12.

3. Northrup, *Women's Wisdom, Women's Bodies*, 231.

4. Donald H. Bell, *Being a Man: The Paradox of Masculinity* (Lexington, Mass.: The Lewis Publishing Company, 1982), 58.

5. Michael S. Kimmel, "Clarence, William, Iron Mike, Tailhook, Senator Packwood, Spur Posse, Magic . . . and Us," in *Transforming a Rape Culture*, Pamela R. Fletcher and Martha Roth, eds. (Minneapolis: Milkweed Editions, 1995), 123-124.

6. Lee Ellis and Linda Ebertz, eds., *Sexual Orientation: Toward Biological Understanding* (Westport, Conn.: Greenwood Publishing Group, Inc./Praeger Publishers), 1997.

7. Diane E. Papalia and Sally Wendkos Olds, *Psychology*, 2nd ed. (New York: McGraw-Hill Book Company, 1985), 441.

8. Papalia and Olds, *Psychology*, 441.

9. Papalia and Olds, *Psychology*, 440.

10. John Leland, "Bisexuality is the wild card of our erotic life. Now it's coming out in the open—in pop culture, in cyberspace and on campus. But can you really have it both ways?" *Newsweek*, July 17, 1995, 47.

11. Stanley M. Aronson, "The Perils of Sexual Ambiguity," Commentary, *The Providence Journal-Bulletin*, May 13, 1996, D-4.

12. Leland, "Bisexuality is the wild card . . . ," 47-48.

13. The AIDS epidemic has created an awareness of the need for health care and preventive measures, especially in the homosexual population, that extends beyond considerations of "safe sex." (AIDS also creates patients, many of whom are male and homosexual but an increasing number of whom are heterosexuals of both genders.) In addition, many activists for gay rights have also become activists for preventive health care. Lesbian activists, in particular, are likely to have ties to broader women's groups and to the still predominantly female self-help movement.

Gay men, meanwhile, tend to be somewhat more image-conscious than their heterosexual counterparts—perhaps because, like heterosexual women, they are seeking to appeal to men, who rely more on visual stimulation than do women. Gays therefore tend to work harder than straight men at keeping themselves in good physical condition. They may consider regular checkups to be a part of their ongoing body-maintenance program.

14. Kimmel, "Clarence, William, Iron Mike, Tailhook, Senator Packwood, Spur Posse, Magic . . . and Us," 123.

15. Kimmel, "Clarence, William, Iron Mike, Tailhook, Senator Packwood, Spur Posse, Magic . . . and Us," 126.

16. Kimmel, "Clarence, William, Iron Mike, Tailhook, Senator Packwood, Spur Posse, Magic . . . and Us," 127-128.

17. Reay Tannahill, *Sex In History* (Chelsea, Miss.: Scarborough House, 1992), 173.

18. Sheldon H. Kardener, Marielle Fuller, and Ivan N. Mensh, "A Survey of Physicians' Attitudes and Practices Regarding Erotic and Nonerotic Contact with Patients," *American Journal of Psychiatry*, 130 (October 1973): 1077.

— 3 —

Touch

How we're touched, when we're touched, where we're touched, who touches us, and what are the reasons for the touch—all of these affect how we respond to touch. It is an individual matter that is based on our being mammals, and primates, and humans, on our gender, on our cultures' attitudes about touch, on our families' attitudes about touch, on our own particular likes and dislikes, and on our particular histories of experience with touch.

Also important is our readiness for touch: Is this a context in which we expect to be touched? Wish to be touched? Are we feeling uneasy? Vulnerable? Needy? Sensual? Have we been getting enough touch lately? These are all factors that influence our response to touch.

"The greatest sense in our body is our touch sense," J. Lionel Taylor wrote in his book *The Stages of Human Life.* "It is probably the chief sense in the processes of sleeping and waking; it gives us our knowledge of depth or thickness and form; we feel, we love and hate, are touchy and are touched, through the touch corpuscles of our skin."[1]

PERCEPTION AND TOUCH

The skin represents much more than just an integument designed to keep the skeleton from falling apart . . . it is in its own right a complex and fascinating organ. In addition to being the largest organ of the body, the various elements comprising the skin have a very large representation in the brain.[2]

The touch sense provides each of us with a tremendous amount of information, but tremendous differences exist in the use we make of it. Ashley Montagu, in his book _Touching: The Human Significance of the Skin_,[3] distinguishes between individuals who are sight-oriented and those who are touch-oriented. The discipline of Neuro-Linguistic Patterning (NLP) adds a third category, "auditory," for individuals who are hearing-oriented. These are the ways in which we receive information; the sources of information on which we rely.

Someone who is primarily touch-oriented, or "kinesthetic" in NLP jargon, will perceive a wider range of subtlety of tactile sensation when touching or being touched than will someone who is primarily visual or auditory. Often this perception is below the level of conscious awareness, so that the individual is left with "feelings" about the experience. If the person who touches him or her is having sexual thoughts and feelings, or has any other hidden agenda, this may be picked up by the individual who is being touched.

Someone who is visually oriented may be especially likely to pick up the corresponding nuances of body language, whether consciously or unconsciously. Likewise, someone who is hearing-oriented, or auditory, may be especially good at reading tone of voice for its conscious and unconscious messages.

But while some of differences in the way and the extent to which we perceive touch may be innate, others may be learned or conditioned. People who are awkward and clumsy in their physical interactions with others may have been raised in a family where there was little touching, or may lacked closeness with one or more of their parents. Such early experiences can affect people for a lifetime.

TOUCH AND GENDER

For men in our society, touch traditionally has been limited almost entirely to violent or sexual encounters. (An exception has been made for athletes and soldiers, among whom a rough yet affectionate contact traditionally has been allowed.) Some men, therefore, may lack a repertoire of non-sexual, non-violent touch, and may not even recognize its existence. To these individuals, every touch is either an attack or a come-on.

For women in our society, touch is a more important part of sexuality, but it is also likely to be a more important part of caring and communication. They are more likely to have, and to expect, a broader repertoire of touch.

Early socialization probably plays a role in these gender differences, which are much less noticeable in other cultures. From birth, babies in our society tend to be given less affectionate touching if they are boys, more if they are girls. And a lack of affectionate touching in infancy and early childhood has been linked with higher rates of violence and aggression in later life.

But as great as the gender differences in early touch may be, they pale beside the differences that are found from one family to another. One family may be very physically demonstrative; in another, days may elapse without any touch between most family members.

TOUCH AND CULTURE

Just as there are *families* in which there is minimal touch, so there are *cultures* in which there is little or no touch. In the United States, this can be seen in the difference between the culture of the North and the South, or in the differences exhibited by members of different ethnic or immigrant groups. The amount of personal space with which people feel comfortable and the amount of eye contact they employ in different situations also vary from culture to culture.

The Japanese strove to maintain, at least through the 1960s, constant contact with their children. Whole families would bathe together. Japanese infants generally received, and continue to receive, a much greater quantity of affectionate touch than do most American infants.

The goal of mothers in the United States is for their children to become active and self-assertive. The goal of Japanese mothers is for their children to be contented and passive. This difference in goals, and in early touch, probably accounts for the difference in activity level between Japanese children and American children. But the difference in the amount of early touch has other implications, as well. "Cultures that show more physical affection toward infants and children tend to have lower rates of adult violence."[4]

Understanding the cultural differences that exist in the use and perception of touch is especially important for doctors, nearly all of whom see—and touch—patients from different cultures.

TOUCH, PROXIMITY, AND INTIMACY

"Touch is the first sense to develop in humans. It may be the last to fade."[5] It affects each of us deeply. It is a creator of intimacy. It is a means of communication. It is a part of many social interactions. But until recent years, the many roles of touch had received little attention from Western science. This is particularly unfortunate given the explosive emotional charge that touch may carry in a society, like ours, where non-sexual touch is a rarity and where any touch can engender feelings of danger.

America is what anthropologists call a "nontactile" society. Compared with most cultures, we are—so to speak—touchy about touch. When psychologist Sidney Jourard observed rates of casual touch among couples in cafés around the world, he reported the highest rate in Puerto Rico (180 times per hour). One of the lowest rates was in the U.S. (two times per hour). [Touch Research Institute psychologist Tiffany] Field has discovered that French parents and children touch each other three times more frequently than their American counterparts, a pattern that continues with age. At McDonald's restaurants in Paris and Miami, Field found that French adolescents demonstrate significantly more casual touching—leaning on a friend, putting an arm around another's shoulder. American teenagers were more likely to fiddle with rings, crack their knuckles and engage in other forms of self-stimulation. "French parents and teachers alike are more physically affectionate and the kids are less aggressive," says Field.[6]

Just the nearness of one person to another—a prerequisite of a physical examination, and of many treatments—creates a sense of artificial intimacy that must be handled with care. This is particularly true in the United States and Canada, where in many regions it is rare for people to come within arm's length of one another in business and social situations.

The amount of "personal space" that people require in order to feel comfortable varies by region, by culture and by situation. In fact, an entire branch of study, called proxemics, is now devoted to evaluating the use of distance in social interactions.

In the Middle East and Latin America, people commonly station themselves within one or two feet of one another, instead of three or four. And in a family setting, or in the anonymity of a crowded bus or stadium, more closeness is tolerated. But in a one-on-one situation, such closeness as is created in a doctor's exam room is rare outside the bedroom. Training in how to handle such professional intimacy is long overdue.

TOUCH BETWEEN DOCTOR AND PATIENT

Touch in the doctor/patient relationship generally involves the patient *giving up* power to the practitioner. Here, however, is the story of a patient who turned the tables, using touch to *take back* power over his own situation:

On the morning after his ten-hour operation, Chuck awoke to a web of tubes. Ominous whispers could be heard outside his room. Then the medieval procession known as grand rounds began, and seven sober residents and interns entered single file and circled his bed, holding clipboards against their chests like dueling shields. Peggy felt violated for her husband—he seemed so vulnerable and exposed—but his first words let her know he was still fighting for control.

Chuck: "You have to understand . . . . Anyone who works on me has to touch me." I reached out to the Chief, who took my hand and held it. With my other hand, I reached for an intern: "That means everybody." Like awkward schoolchildren, they looked to their Chief for permission.

[An intern stepped forward, introduced himself, and touched Chuck.]

Chuck: "Good, that may be the best medicine you'll ever dispense."[7]

Touch is a way of showing concern. And touch is a form of communication. These qualities of touch can allow for closer connections in the doctor/patient relationship—when touch is used appropriately, and with awareness and consent on the part of the patient.

As health professionals, we may find ourselves in a position where we are tempted to compensate for our patients' lack of satisfactory or sufficient early touch. And, if our own early touch experiences were not satisfactory or sufficient, we may also feel a need to compensate for that lack in some way. As Touch Research Institute psychologist Tiffany Field has put it, "America is suffering from an epidemic of skin hunger."[8] But a practice setting is not the place to satisfy that hunger; attempting to do so can be highly dangerous.

Procedures requiring touching of patients are very vulnerable to misinterpretation. Ensuring that patients understand at all times what is being done, and why, will greatly reduce the risk of offence. Deft, careful touching of patients will reduce also the likelihood of avoidable pain and will encourage the patient to relax and cooperate in ways that will save time and produce better results.[9]

Doctors would benefit greatly from educating themselves about the aspects of touch that can affect the doctor/patient relationship. It is for this reason that we have devised the Safe Touch Protocol (see Part III of this book).

What do doctors need to know about touching a patient? Whenever we reach out to touch patients, there are a number of points to consider:

- Good intentions are not enough.
- You may never know how the use of touch in a patient's family, and in the patient's culture, has shaped his or her perception of touch.
- You may never learn about a patient's history with other doctors, positive or negative.
- Your own family and cultural background will have a bearing on how comfortable you are with touching others, and on how others will perceive your touching.
- You will be affected by—but may not be aware of—your own needs regarding touch at the time at which you are seeing the patient.

All of this will have a bearing on how comfortable you will be with touch and on how comfortably your touch will be perceived by your patients.

But remember, some of our most intimate times involve being touched, so when a person is touched by someone who he or she barely knows, some unusual reactions can be expected.

Because we will rarely know the specifics of any patient's past experiences, we will need to use all of our verbal and nonverbal skills to assess our patient's needs. By employing sufficient sensitivity, we will be enabled to make an educated assessment of how to proceed with touching each individual.

We also need to be very aware of the skills and attitudes that we bring to touch. When we touch, we give very clear messages—including some messages of which we are aware, and some of which we are not.

Kinds of Touch

There are many kinds of touch, many perceptions of touch, many ways to touch, and many intentions in touching. Some are appropriate in the doctor/ patient relationship, and some are inappropriate.

· All health-care professionals who touch patients would be wise to be aware of the power of touch. Since there are many kinds of touch, ways of touching, and ways of perceiving the touch that is received, it is not always possible to predict what the effects of touch will be.

Perceptions of Touch. Each instance of touch will be perceived by the individual being touched as having certain qualities: firm, soft, hard, painful, gentle, soothing, rough, careless, sensitive, insensitive, assertive, dominating, submissive, half-hearted, tentative, assured, deliberate, icky, wishy-washy, clammy, gripping, prodding, poking, unwilling, jabbing, jolting, cold, warm, passionate, respectful, disrespectful, trembling, uncertain, stroking, hesitant, groping.

Intentions of Touch. Note that the doctor's *intention* may be very different from the patient's *perception*. If the intention is strictly procedural, but the patient feels that he or she has been improperly cared for, you may have a serious communication problem and you may even have a lawsuit on your hands (see Informed Consent, in Chapter 6, "How Misconduct Occurs"). Examples of appropriate and inappropriate qualities of touch are presented in Table 3.1.

Table 3.1
Doctor/Patient Touch

Appropriate Qualities: Respecting doctor/patient boundaries	Inappropriate Qualities: Violating doctor/patient boundaries
comforting	sexual
caring	insensitive
deft	clumsy
procedural	haphazard
healing	hurtful
supportive	brusque

Uses of Touch. Just as they may assume that their patients' perception of a touch is the same as their intention of touch, many practitioners assume that they *know* what effect their use of touch may have on their patients—but, again, many of them are wrong. For example, a chiropractor in Ontario reports that he used to routinely pat his patients on the rear to signal that he wanted them to turn over—until a patient told him how she had left another chiropractor because he did that. That was a rude awakening for the practitioner, but not nearly so rude as a lawsuit would have been.

When asked about their experiences with doctor/patient touch, patients were quick to complain of cold hands and cold instruments, especially if either had been wielded by a gynecologist, urologist, or proctologist. Some spoke of being startled by practitioners who, while out of sight of the patient, gave no warning of their intentions. One told of an orthopaedist who didn't know when to quit: The doctor's forceful examination of an injured knee was causing the patient a great deal of pain. "Stop. Stop it. Stop that, right now," the patient demanded. But that demand was neither heeded nor acknowledged until the patient—by now, in tears—bellowed "Stop, or I'll sue!"

Some patients described behavior that was decidedly inappropriate. One patient told of a physician who never mentioned an antibiotic without discussing its efficacy for venereal diseases, and whose crotch pressed against the patient whenever the doctor measured blood pressure, listened to chest sounds, or peered into a sore throat. Despite the many free samples, that doctor now has at least one less patient. Another patient talked about a chiropractor who was competent, cute, charming, and friendly—a little too friendly. At first, the jokes and chit-chat were comforting, the patient recalled. But by the third or fourth visit, things seemed a little too intense, "almost like he was flirting with me," and she began to become uneasy around him. One day, as she lay face-down on the table, he tickled her with the tip of her long braid. "What did he think he was doing? " she said. "He's supposed to be a professional. And the way he kept looking at me and talking to me . . . . I think he was flirting with me. What am I saying? I know he was flirting with me. I just didn't want to believe it. He *was* flirting with me. And I don't like it."

Several other patients spoke of problems with touch that, though also inappropriate, they believed to have been accidental. One woman told of the gynecologist whom she abandoned after a single pelvic exam, during which the doctor was all thumbs, and those thumbs kept bumping painfully against her clitoris. Two others described problems with dentists or orthodontists who—while working in their patients' mouths—failed to keep sufficient track of their own arms. Both women mentioned the discomfort and embarrassment they had felt as the dentists' elbows or forearms repeatedly brushed their breasts.

It can be valuable to ask yourself questions like these: How do my patients perceive my touch? How do they feel about my use of touch? Am I using touch in ways that make people uncomfortable? Could I alter my touching in any way to ensure that more of my patients will feel comfortable?

Feedback about Touch

Sources of such information can include direct or indirect patient comments to you or your staff. This feedback could be very indirect; for example, whether a patient returns, or whether a patient refers other people to you. An anonymous survey can be very helpful in soliciting more direct feedback. A patient questionnaire and sample cover letter for current and former patients are included in Chapter 13, the "Safe Practice Analysis"—a part of the Practice Protection Protocol that is presented in Part III of this book.

Negative feedback can be difficult to deal with. But when you know how patients truly feel, you will have the opportunity to assess yourself and to make any necessary changes. This is far superior to merely wondering or assuming. To make procedural touch safer and more comfortable for both doctor and patient, we have created guidelines for safe touching. These can be found in Chapter 12, the "Safe Touch Protocol," in Part III of this book.

Effects of Gender and Sexuality

Substantial gender differences have been found in the use of touch and proximity in the health-care relationship. Men in our society have been socialized to see touching as a means of obtaining sex or enforcing power; this discourages the use of casual touch in conversation. They may see proximity as a threat to their autonomy, and eye contact as a challenge to their dominance; this discourages the use of either in non-confrontational situations. Women, on the other hand, have been socialized to think of touching as a means of conveying support or sympathy; they use more touching in their conversations. They have been socialized to see proximity and eye contact as means of establishing a valuable interpersonal connection; they therefore are likely to be comfortable with more eye-contact and closer interpersonal distances. Not surprisingly, male doctor/ male patient interactions have been found to involve the least amount of touching, the lowest level of eye contact and the widest interpersonal distances.[10]

These are only generalities, however. The reality is that attitudes toward touch, proximity and eye contact vary more from culture to culture, or family to family, than from gender to gender. They are shaped by genetics and early childhood experiences, and are influenced by the events of a lifetime. There is no substitute, therefore, for careful observation of the patient's responses.

Touch, Connection, and Power

When a patient is seeking to connect with the practitioner, then more eye contact and a somewhat closer interpersonal distance may be helpful. When a patient is feeling threatened, less eye contact, an indirect posture (that is, not facing the person straight-on), and a greater distance may be helpful.

A belligerent patient may be reacting to a perceived threat to his or her autonomy; try making eye contact while asking questions, then looking at your clipboard and making notes while the patient responds. Some timid patient will be drawn out by a friendly approach that establishes a rapport, while others will respond better to an impersonal approach that minimizes the power differential.

It is vital to make any procedure involving touch as comfortable and as safe as possible for doctor and patient. The process will always be one of trial and error, but training and experience will help to minimize the amount of error.

NOTES

1. J. Lionel Taylor, excerpt from his landmark book, *The Stages of Human Life*,

as quoted in *Touching: The Human Significance of the Skin*, by Ashley Montagu (New York: Columbia University Press, 1971), 157.

2. Ashley Montagu, *Touching: The Human Significance of the Skin* (New York: Columbia University Press, 1971), 6.

3. Montagu, *Touching*.

4. George Howe Colt, with reporting by Anne Hollister, "The Magic of Touch: Massage's Healing Powers Make it Serious Medicine," *Life* (August 1997), 62.

5. Colt, "The Magic of Touch," 62.

6. Colt, "The Magic of Touch," 60-62.

7. Gail Sheehy, *New Passages: Mapping Your Life Across Time* (New York: Random House, 1995), 165.

8. Colt, "The Magic of Touch," 62.

9. *Prevention of Sexual Abuse of Patients: Introductory Instructor's Guide for Diploma Programs in Medical Radiation Technology* (Toronto, Ontario, Canada: College of Medical Radiation Technologists of Ontario, 1994), 13.

10. Debra L. Roter and Judith A. Hall, *Doctors Talking With Patients/Patients Talking With Doctors: Improving Communication in Medical Visits* (Westport, Conn.: Auburn House, 1992), 63.

— *4* —

Explorations and Applications

Gender, sexuality and touch in the doctor/patient relationship are issues that have always affected both doctor and patient, yet until recently, they have been little touched-upon in the education of physicians. All health-care practitioners need training in these areas, training that involves looking at their attitudes and behaviors regarding gender, sexuality, and touch. Until these subjects become a standard part of doctor education, doctors will be more likely to care for their patients in ways that are inappropriate and even harmful, in ways that are at odds with the very purpose of health care.

PERSONAL EXPLORATIONS IN GENDER, SEXUALITY, AND TOUCH

It is important to acknowledge that we all have limiting ideas and ingrained biases that affect our perceptions. Figuring out what these ideas and biases are, and maintaining an awareness of what affects they might have, is the key to dealing with them rationally and appropriately. For instance, if you feel uncomfortable in the presence of a certain patient, it is helpful to understand why.

Gender
1. What is your gender identity? Is it predominately what our society currently categorizes as masculine or feminine? How do you feel about that?
2. What range of gender roles are you comfortable with in others?
    a. Do you feel comfortable around a very businesslike woman?
    b. Do you feel comfortable around a very nurturing man?
3. Do you appreciate someone who can comfortably shift from one gender role to another—in other words, with someone who has a wide personality range?
4. How satisfying do you find your relationship with your female patients? With your male patients?
5. What percentage of your female patients do you believe are satisfied with you

as a doctor? How many would say so to your face? On an anonymous questionnaire?

6. What is the percentage of male and female patients in your practice? Why do you think that is? Is it because of your gender? Your level of comfort with a certain gender? Your circle of contacts?

7. Do you prefer caring for female patients? For male patients? Why?

8. How would you characterize your average male patients? your average female patients? What are your relationships generally like with each?

9. How would you rate yourself as a health-care provider for female patients and male patients, in terms of respect, sensitivity, flexibility, openness, and being non-judgmental?

10. What changes do you think you might need to make in the way you care for male patients? For female patients?

11. What kind of training or help will you need to make those changes?

Discussion. If you are a man, you may still have characteristics that would be considered feminine in our culture—for example, nurturing and sensitivity. If you are a woman, you may have qualities generally considered masculine—for example, independence and intellectualism. Just being a man or a woman does not mean that you must adopt the roles generally prescribed for that gender. A mix of gender traits can create a balanced, more successful personality. It also can create a balanced, more successful physician. Besides, we all should have the choice to be ourselves.

Sexuality

1. How would you describe your views regarding sexuality? As liberal? Moderate? Conservative? Extreme?

2. How would you describe your personal sexual practices, or your beliefs regarding sexual practices?

3. How do you feel about what others do sexually, and with whom?

4. Do you believe that everyone should believe and behave as you do?

5. What fantasies do you have that you would like fulfilled? Do you have fantasies involving any of your patients?

6. Are your sexual beliefs, fantasies, or practices ever a problem for you in your practice? How so?

7. Are your patient's beliefs, fantasies, or practices—as evident in how they act, what they tell you, or in what you suspect—ever a problem for you? How so?

8. Do you ever try to impose your ideas on your patients? on your staff?

9. What changes do you think you may need to make, to care for both male and female patients more appropriately?

10. What might you need to learn about sexuality in general, and about your own sexuality in particular?

Discussion. It is important to be aware of your own sexuality and sexual impulses because repressing such feelings does not make them go away. Consciously or unconsciously, they will affect your actions. This does not mean going through the day thinking, ''What a fox,'' or ''What I wouldn't do to get a piece of that action!'' Rather, it may mean thinking, "I'm somewhat attracted to this patient; I'll have to be especially careful.''

It also is important to be aware of your sexual attitudes and biases, because only then can you prevent them from interfering with patient care. As a doctor, you have a duty to set aside your own interest and agendas, and act only in the interest of your patients.

Touch

1. What is your family background regarding touch?
   a. Was there a lot of touching?
   b. Was there very little or no touching?
   c. Were you made to feel bad about touching yourself?
   d. What ideas does your family of origin have regarding touch?
2. What are your beliefs and practices regarding touch?
3. What effect do your beliefs and practices regarding touch have on your practice?
4. Do you find yourself enjoying touching much more with some of your patients than with others?
5. Do your background and your beliefs leave you feeling deprived of touch?
6. Do you get much touch in your personal life and social interactions?
7. What effect do your patient's beliefs regarding touch have on them?
8. Do you ever find yourself focusing on getting your needs met, while you are touching your patients?
9. Do you find yourself focusing your attention on what your patients needs are regarding touch?
10. How would you rate your sensitivity to patients in matters of touch?
11. What changes do you feel you may need to make concerning touching patients?
12. What do you need to learn about touch and the doctor/patient relationship?

Discussion. Touch is a powerful sense that conveys much information—whether or not there is a conscious understanding on the part of the toucher or the touched of the message being conveyed. In a low-touch society, such as ours, each touch that does occur is much more potent.

Both doctors and patients may have a limited vocabulary of touch. They may lack a social framework for non-violent, non-sexual touch. Doctors and patients with touch-deprived personal lives may have an unrecognized craving for affectionate or sexual touch. They may seek to satisfy this craving in an inappropriate setting, such as the doctor's office, in which case they are likely to rationalize and justify behavior that they themselves do not really understand.

Particular care must be taken, therefore, to ensure that examinations and procedures involving touch are handled in a manner that is asexual and unthreatening. The keys to this are gaining an understanding of your own motivations, finding appropriate ways of filling your own needs for touch, and expanding your touch vocabulary.

PRACTICAL APPLICATIONS FOR PRACTITIONERS

Learning more about your patients and yourself can be enriching in and of itself. But it also has great practical value. It can help you communicate more efficiently and effectively with your patients. It can reduce the likelihood of your giving offense. It can improve your relationship with your patients, so that you get fewer complaints and more referrals. These tips are just a beginning.

Gender

Some recommendations for doctor/patient interactions are the same for patients of either gender: Avoid broad comments about males and females. Avoid stereotypical thinking and behavior. Avoid any behavior that is likely to be considered offensive. Be prepared for patients to stereotype you.

When Working with Male Patients. Draw them out; encourage them; educate them. Because male patients may communicate less, you cannot assume that they have understood everything or that they have informed you of everything you need to know.

1. Be sure you understand their condition and concerns. Male patients generally ask fewer questions, and in some cases, men won't even ask a question unless they think they know the answer. Some may be like the former fighter pilot who used to refuse to ask questions of his physician, saying, "He doesn't tell me how to fly a plane. I don't tell him how to be a doctor."[1]

2. Be sure nothing important is left out. Male patients may be reluctant to volunteer information, assuming that if it were important, you would ask. Pay close attention to body language, tone, and facial expression for signs of something you haven't been told, or for unspoken reservations. Once you do get them talking, hear them out; if you interrupt or cut them off, you are likely to miss important diagnostic clues and information about their treatment goals.

3. Be sure your explanations and instructions are understood. Pay close attention to body language, tone, and facial expression for signs that all the information you are giving is being understood. Since male patients may feel a need to have all the answers, and a need to be able to fix things themselves, they may see having to ask you questions as a sign of failure. Ask male patients to repeat instructions, to be certain that they understood. Listen carefully to their responses. Repeat and restate your instructions or explanations as necessary, until you are certain they have been understood.

4. Generally, be encouraging. Congratulate your male patients for following through with instructions and taking care of themselves. Encourage them to come in for checkups and care.

5. Be on the lookout for the strong, silent syndrome. Watch for "hero" characteristics—the "I can handle it and I'm just fine the way I am" syndrome. Trying to be like John Wayne or Clint Eastwood has its price:

   a. Men are less likely to look for early warning signs of illness. They may not know how to do self-exams, such as checking for signs of testicular cancer.

   b. Men more often engage in dangerous and high-stress professions.

   c. They often wait to report an illness or injury until it results in an actual loss of function.

6. Allow more personal space. Men are less comfortable sitting face-to-face with someone in a therapeutic situation. When dealing with strangers, they generally prefer a greater interpersonal distance than women from the same culture. Consider sitting or standing further away during discussions with your male patients, and coming close only during procedures.

7. Limit eye contact. Many men regard prolonged eye contact as threatening. They tend to be more talkative when they can't see the person they're talking to. You may get more information from such patients if you do not try to face them all the time, but speak less directly. What is more, gaze plays a leading role in courtship rituals. So when a woman looks at a man, or a man at a woman, the recipient of the gaze may assume that it is an indication of sexual interest.

8. Limit touch. Though this is less true for more-recent generations, men in our society tend to regard touch as either sexual or violent. They therefore may be uncomfortable with same-sex touching, and may be too comfortable with opposite-sex touching.

9. Limit power. Men are usually more comfortable sharing intimate details with a woman, but decidedly less so when they are confronted by someone of greater authority than themselves. To draw them out, it may be necessary to shift to a less-powerful, less-threatening doctoring style.

10. Beware of stereotypes. But doctors and patients alike must exercise caution in dealing with men who have not worked through their prejudices.

When Working with Female Patients. Listen to them; relate to them; connect with them.

1. Remember, all smiles aren't equal. Women typically smile more often, even when saying negative things and when being aggressive, whereas men are likely to smile only when saying something positive. This is not hypocrisy on the part of women, but a typical primate behavior. It reflects an attempt—probably unconscious—by someone in a lower-status position to avoid angering a higher-status individual.

2. Be caring. Women are more relationship-oriented than men; they are likely to want a more personal relationship with a care-giver. They are likely to tolerate closer proximity and to expect more eye contact.

3. Give feedback. Women are more likely to seek and to expect confirmation that they have been heard and understood.

4. Don't cut them off. Doctors of either gender are more likely to interrupt their female patients. But if you don't hear them out, you are likely to miss important diagnostic clues and information about their treatment goals.

5. Expect questions; have answers. Women are more likely to have questions and comments. They also are more likely to follow through on treatment decisions—especially if they have participated in making them.

6. Expect proactivity. Women tend to be more aware of health issues—and not just for themselves. They often act as their families' gatekeepers for health care.
   a. They are more likely to know about and perform self-examinations.
   b. They are more likely to be recognize to the first signs of a problem, and they are more likely to seek treatment before a problem becomes serious.
   c. They are more likely to schedule checkups and routine exams.

7. Be sure you are understood. Some women may be too intimidated, especially

during a discussion that is held when they are only semi-clothed, to question your instructions or explanations. Others may be too proud. Men aren't the only ones who try to be strong and silent.

8. Don't trivialize. There is a general tendency on the part of doctors, male and female, to take women's complaints less seriously; be very careful not to do so.

9. Don't stereotype. Stereotypical thinking is likely to get you into hot water, as women are particularly likely to be sensitive to these kinds of attitudes. Instead, be prepared for a wide range of behavior from female patients.

For Male or Female Patients. If a patient is exhibiting behavior that is more common in people of the other gender, switch tactics. For instance, draw out silent women. Encourage timid men. Avoid eye contact with people who it seems to anger or intimidate. Limit proximity to what seems comfortable for that particular patient.

Touch
1. Be sensitive. If you are the touchy-feely type, consider altering your behavior around patients. Some people are not comfortable with being touched, though they may try to be polite about it.

2. Be skillful. If you know that your touch is sensual or sexual, or too tentative, or too rough, or you've gotten that feedback from some people, practice different kinds of touch. Expand your touch repertoire.

3. Be sure you have consent. Make it a habit to prepare patients for where, when, and why you'll be touching them.

4. Avoid hugging. If you initiate hugs, you may be forcing yourself on patients, making them uncomfortable, or using your position of power to get your own needs met. Hugging patients can also begin a pattern of more and more intimacies; therefore, consider doing very little hugging of patients, or none at all.

5. Be careful. Is helping your patients always your only goal when you touch them? Whose needs are being met?

6. Avoid casual touch. Touch that is not a necessary part of a diagnostic or therapeutic procedure can easily be misused, misinterpreted or misunderstood. Be aware of when, how, and whom you touch casually.

7. Be prepared to be touched. Your patients may also use touch. Be aware of their touch and what it might mean.

Sexuality
1. Be restrained. If you are a very sexual person, you may want to consider toning that down in the office. But be sure you continue to monitor your thoughts and behaviors—do not ignore them.

2. Be polite. If you are frank about sexuality, could that ever be offensive?

3. Avoid disparaging remarks. It is easy to give offense. You can never be certain who's in your office, or what a given person's background might be.

4. Avoid bias. Does a different sexual orientation from yours make you uncomfortable? Why is that? Do you send those vibes to your patients?

5. Avoid sexual jokes. Someone may laugh or seem to go along with your jokes, yet not like them; it could be that the person feels offended but is trying to be polite.

6. Avoid sexually charged terms. Such terms, however lightly intended, can also be a problem. Using slang terms for body parts or biological functions can sexualize the doctor/patient relationship. Use their proper names when possible—though explanations may sometimes be required. Avoid expressions such as "get your butt over here."

Attractions

1. If you sense that a patient has an interest in you, remember, the attraction may be less to you than to your role as a care-giver. People like to be taken care of. (See Transference and Countertransference, in Chapter 9, "The Doctor Role.")

Also, be especially meticulous about your record-keeping with this patient. Record the reason for and outcome of every procedure, and be sure to make not of any odd or disturbing comments or behavior.

2. If you have an interest in a patient, think. Ask yourself, If there are so many people out there, why am I finding myself so attracted to a patient? Am I spending too much time in the office, and too little socializing? What's really going on?

3. If emotions start running high and the doctor/patient relationship starts to break down, get help.

4. If in doubt, refer the patient to someone else.

5. Whenever dealing with an attraction to a patient:

    a. Consider the possible effect on the patient.

    b. Consider the possible effects on you and your practice.

    d. Take good notes of everything that transpires between you.

    c. Understand that simply dismissing the patient does not clear you of any responsibility.

    e. If necessary, contact your licensing board and ask its advice.

    f. If you both care for each other, discharge the patient, and do not have *any* contact for a period of at least six months. (This is the minimum time for doctors, in most areas, unless they undergo counseling. Psychiatrists are generally required to allow a two-year period between treating and dating, if indeed they ever date former patients.) When that time is up, the two of you can determine whether you both still have an interest in one another, and if so, can begin dating then. Ideally, check this situation out with a supervisor/buddy.

6. Always consider the risks. Are you really willing to lose everything? Your practice? Your property? Your reputation?

NOTE

1. Several iatrogenic illnesses later, this gentleman no longer hesitates to question his physicians. He has become much more of an partner in his own health-care team. He also has become much healthier. In general, the squeaky wheel gets better care.

PART II

Sexual Misconduct

And we must remember: any form of abuse that comes from the very people who are supposed to protect us, to whom we have no choice but to make ourselves vulnerable, is the most destructive of self.

—*Gloria Steinem,*
"Revolution from Within," 1992

— 5 —

What Is Misconduct?

The number of sexual misconduct complaints against health-care professionals is increasing at an alarming rate. A 1992 study by the Federation of State Medical Boards reported charges that year against 132 medical doctors in 42 states, compared with charges in 1990 against 84 doctors in 35 states—and the tide of complaints continues to rise. Of those medical doctors whose cases received formal board action, approximately half lost their licenses to practice their profession.[1] A 1994 study by the Federation of Chiropractic Licensing Boards likewise found that, across North America, misconduct complaints against chiropractors also are on the rise.[2]

These allegations of sexual misconduct are creating casualties on all sides: doctors who lose their licenses, practices, or reputations; patients who are traumatized by inappropriate or abusive behavior, or behavior that they perceive as abusive; and health-care professions that are publicly humiliated or singled out for unflattering media attention.

A FIDUCIARY FAILURE

Sexual misconduct is, to say the least, a very complex problem. It encompasses issues of sex, gender, power, and communication, as well as, in some cases, a real pathology on the part of the health-care professional.

Sexual misconduct occurs when the fiduciary aspect of the health-care relationship is compromised. "Fiduciary" is a legal term that is applied to a professional in whom a client (in this case, the patient) places his or her trust. Because such professionals are in positions of power relative to their clients, the law holds them to a higher standard of behavior. They are required to place the interests of their clients above and before their own. A comprehensive, even exhaustive, exploration of this and related topics is presented in the book *Sexual*

Abuse by Professionals: A Legal Guide.[3]

All health-care professionals have a fiduciary relationship with their patients. In other words, the professional is in a position of power, while the patient is in a position of weakness and vulnerability. Although the patient may not be directly aware of the power imbalance, the professional is nonetheless obligated to understand and control its limits.

AN ANCIENT TRANSGRESSION

The problem of sexual misconduct has been with us for centuries. It was addressed by the Greek physician Hippocrates in the fourth or fifth century B.C., in the Hippocratic Oath that some members of the medical profession continue to use today: "Whatever houses I may visit, I will come for the benefit of the sick, remaining free of all intentional injustice, of all mischief, and in particular, of sexual relationships with both female and male persons."[4]

Similar admonishments to doctors, warning them against inappropriate sexual behavior toward their patients, have been found in European medical texts from the Middle Ages and Renaissance.

AN EQUAL OPPORTUNITY PROBLEM

Statistics on the subject reveal that approximately seventy percent of sexual misconduct complaints against health professionals, psychotherapists, and clergy are filed by female patients or clients against male professionals. Approximately twenty percent are from female patients or clients complaining about female professionals. Of the remaining ten percent of complaints, roughly five percent are from male patients or clients complaining about men, and the remaining five percent are from male patients or clients bringing allegations against women. Females, therefore, make up about ninety percent of the victims of sexual misconduct, and twenty-five percent of the alleged perpetrators.[5] It should be noted, however, that many of those working in the field "have speculated that male victims of professionals of either gender are underrepresented across the board because of particular male characteristics inhibiting both recognition and reporting [of abuse]."[6]

Female doctors may think they are immune to complaints of misconduct, but the statistics prove them wrong. What is more, women may be especially at risk from the very obsessive patient. The patient behavior that tends to be the most obsessive is that which occurs between a female patient and a female doctor.[7]

BREAKING THE SILENCE

Patients used to keep silent about improper behavior, but that is rapidly changing. Now, patients are speaking out in record numbers—and this is only the beginning.

Until very recently, the complaint process has been little-known, little-used, and far from impartial. To quote the organizers of the Third International Conference on Sexual Exploitation by Health Professionals, Psychotherapists and Clergy, "The tendency is to shoot the messenger, blame the victim and coddle the man."[8] However, as patients become less afraid of complaining, as awareness of the complaint process rises, and as the complaint process itself becomes fairer and less humiliating for the person filing charges, the number of complaints can be expected to continue its dramatic increase.

As things now stand, it is up to clients and patients to monitor the behavior and the regulation of practitioners; and it is through their complaints that this monitoring takes place. Women, especially, have become increasingly sensitive to inappropriate or "old-style" behavior on the part of either male or female doctors. In the doctor's office, as in the greater society, they have taken the lead in the fight against abuse, misconduct, and harassment.

The unequal relationship between doctor and patient has taken a tremendous toll, and those patients with the least power in our society—primarily, women, children, and members of ethnic and racial minorities—have been its principal victims. The professionals whose power now is being eroded by increasing scrutiny and regulation may not like the message, but shooting the messenger is hardly the answer.

Widespread educational changes are necessary to prevent a substantial percentage of the next generation of health practitioners from compromising their patients' welfare and the public trust. In some places, that training already has begun. As for the current health professionals whose education included no training in touch, gender, sexuality, communication and other important skills— it is never too late to learn.

What is more, in an increasingly consumerist health-care market, embracing the skills of the new practitioner can bring benefits not only of prevention but also of profit. Those doctors who develop a strong awareness of their own attitudes and behavior; cultivate a wide range of skills in interpersonal communication; and adopt office procedures that protect their patients, especially their female patients, will be far more likely to become or remain successful—as well as to prevent unnecessary difficulties for themselves and their patients.

SEXUAL MISCONDUCT vs. SEXUAL HARASSMENT

What's the Difference?

Both sexual misconduct and sexual harassment can create significant problems in a health-care practice. The two issues are not identical, but they are closely related: Each can be thought of as a boundary violation, occurring when one person's "safe space" is invaded by another.

Sexual Misconduct. This involves the behavior of a doctor or other health-care professional toward a patient or patients. (Sexual misconduct also is an issue in other professions where a fiduciary relationship exists between the professionals and their clients.) An understanding of this issue is vital to all doctors and other health-care professionals.

The boundary violations that constitute physician sexual misconduct do not necessarily involve sexual intercourse between doctor and patient. Inappropriate talk or touching, or unnecessary examinations or treatments, also can qualify.

The laws and professional regulations regarding sexual misconduct are still in a state of flux. But for a hint as to where they are likely to go, it is possible to examine the more fully evolved body of law and regulations relating to sexual harassment. (The nature, causes, and consequences of sexual misconduct in the doctor/patient relationship are further discussed in the remainder of Part II, in Chapters 6 through 10.)

Sexual Harassment. This generally involves the behavior of a supervisor, manager, employer, or employee toward staff at the same or a lower level of power. An understanding of this issue also is vital to all doctors, with the possible exception of those in solo practice who have no staff.

Sexual harassment is an issue arising in a work place or an educational institution. It generally involves one person having power over another's employment, money, grades, or advancement, and abusing that power, though sometimes it instead involves harassment by a co-worker. There are two recognized forms of sexual harassment:

1.   *quid pro quo*: a demand for sexual favors in exchange for job benefits;
2.   a hostile work environment: unwelcome acts such as physical or verbal conduct, or visual displays, that make the individual's job difficult.

The U.S. Equal Employment Opportunity Commission (EEOC) defines sexual harassment as "unwelcome sexual advances, requests for sexual favors and other verbal or physical conduct of a sexual nature" when:

1.   submission to such conduct is made a term or condition of an individual's employment, either implicitly or explicitly;
2.   submission to or rejection of such conduct is used as the basis for employment decisions affecting such individual;
3.   such conduct has the purpose or effect of unreasonably interfering with an individual's work performance or creating an intimidating, offensive, or hostile work environment.

Harassment can come in the form of physical abuse, such as touching, hugging, and stroking. It can come in the form of verbal abuse, which may include inappropriate ways of addressing a person, use of sexually explicit language, or use of words that refer to an individual's body parts. Harassment can involve visual abuse, such as displaying "girlie" or "hunk" calendars or other visually offensive material, regardless of whether that material is intended to offend. The intent of actions such as these generally is difficult to determine.

But a determination of intent is not necessary to a finding of sexual harassment. In cases where it *can* be established that there was an intent to offend, heavier penalties may be exacted.

A finding of *quid pro quo* sexual harassment requires that a plaintiff prove that receiving job benefits or protection from job detriments was dependent upon his or her submission to a supervisor's *unwelcome* sexual demands.

Claims of a hostile work environment generally require that the plaintiff demonstrate not one offensive incident, but a pattern of offensive behavior—unless the one incident was especially outrageous. A single use of offensive language, or a single hug or bump in the hallway, is not sufficient. A hostile work environment claim must prove two things: (1) subjectively, the individual had to regard the behavior as sexual harassment; and (2) another reasonable person would also regard this incident or behavior as sexual harassment.[9]

(The "reasonable person" measure has been modified somewhat in recent years in recognition of the fact that some material, speech, or behavior that is considered outrageous by most women is regarded as acceptable by many men. Instead of a "reasonable person," therefore, a "reasonable woman" standard has been used by the courts in some male-female harassment cases.)

An institution's liability can be established where the employer is found to have had direct or constructive notice of any of these types of sexual harassment and failed to take immediate and appropriate action. Some of the factors that have been considered by courts and enforcement agencies in determining liability are the nature of the conduct, the frequency and openness of the conduct, and whether it could easily have been avoided by the victim.

One longstanding question about sexual harassment recently has been answered: In a March 4, 1998, decision, the U.S. Supreme Court unanimously ruled "that federal law protects employees from being sexually harassed in the workplace by people of the same sex."[10]

Because harassment law has been built on the foundation of the gender-based discrimination clause of Title VII of the Civil Rights Act of 1964, legal authorities had disagreed on whether same-sex behavior could qualify. "Many federal lower courts have either flatly rejected same-sex harassment claims, or have limited them to cases in which a heterosexual employee complains of harassment by a homosexual co-worker. . . . [But] Justice Antonin Scalia said it was the conduct itself, and not the sex or motivation of the people involved, that determined whether sexual harassment amounted to 'discrimination because of sex' . . . . Sexual desire, whether heterosexual or homosexual, was not a necessary element of such a case, he said."[11]

What Are the Similarities?

Abuse of Power. Sexual misconduct and sexual harassment are similar in that each generally involves a person of greater power taking advantage of a person of lesser power. "Sexual harassment is particularly volatile because it often fuses two levels of power: the power of employers over employees and the power of men over women. . . . It is the confusion of public and private, bringing together two arenas of men's power over women. Not only are men in positions of power in the workplace, but we are socialized to be the sexual initiators and to see sexual prowess as a confirmation of masculinity,'' writes Michael Kimmel of SUNY Stonybrook, a sociologist, prolific author, and leader in the field of men's studies.[12] His words about male-female sexual harassment apply just as well to male-female sexual misconduct.

Such abuses of power used to go unnoticed, for the most part, except by their victims. They were borne in silent shame, or were even considered acceptable. In the last few decades, however, that has begun to change. More and more, those who have been abused or wrongfully treated are coming forward.

Possible Absence of Intent. Sexual misconduct and sexual harassment also are similar in that each often arises out of a lack of awareness of what kinds of behavior are offensive or even harmful. As a result, preventive measures for sexual misconduct and sexual harassment also are quite similar: We all need to learn ways of prevention that will safeguard those people with whom we work and those with whom we are involved in health-care relationships.

PREVENTION STRATEGIES

The strategies for preventing either sexual harassment or sexual misconduct include getting training to facilitate an understanding of the power of roles; gaining an understanding of the impact of one's own sexuality and the sexuality of those with whom one interacts professionally; learning appropriate ways of behaving around and of communicating with people of the same gender and of opposite genders; learning what behaviors are considered unacceptable; learning about the situations that may lead up to such transgressions; learning about the effects of abuse and harassment; and understanding the potential legal and financial consequences of unacceptable behavior.

Preventing Sexual Harassment

Here are five specific steps that health-care professionals can take to help sexual harassment by supervisors or co-workers:[13]

1. develop and post a policy against harassment;
2. teach employees what constitutes harassment;
3. improve morale and productivity;
4. address complaints before they develop into litigation;
5. establish an effective and confidential complaint process.

Preventing Sexual Misconduct

Here are five specific steps that health-care professionals can take to help prevent sexual misconduct by care-givers:[14]

1. develop and post a Patient's Bill of Rights;
2. teach yourself and your staff what behavior is unacceptable;
3. improve rapport and communication with patients;
4. address patient complaints and dissatisfaction promptly, before they develop into litigation;
5. a) establish an effective and confidential complaint process; this is an option primarily for hospitals, for other large health-care organizations, and for state or national professional associations and the organizations that regulate them; b) or, for individuals and small-group practices, establish checks and balances on your own behavior and attitudes; for doctors, this could include obtaining feedback on your doctoring techniques. (For help in assessing and altering the way you practice, see Part III, the Patient Protection Protocol.)

NOTES

1. "Tangled Case of Sexual Molestation Pits a Doctor Against 8 Poor Women," *The New York Times*, National Edition, Jan. 29, 1995.

2. Wendy Caro and Angelica Redleaf, "1994 Survey of Licensing Boards in Mexico, Canada, the United States and the Caribbean," conducted for and distributed by the Federation of Chiropractic Licensing Boards (unpublished results).

3. Steven B. Bisbing, Linda Mabus Jorgenson, and Pamela K. Sutherland, *Sexual Abuse by Professionals: A Legal Guide* (Charlottesville, Va.: *Michie*, 1995).

4. From "The Hippocratic Oath," a translation by Ludwig Edelstein that is No. 1 of the *Supplements to the Bulletins of the History of Medicine* (Baltimore: Johns Hopkins University Press, 1943).

5. Comments made by Gary R. Schoener, in "Assessment, Treatment and Supervision of the Professional Offender," a seminar presented by Schoener and John Gonsiorek, at *It's Never O.K., The Third International Conference on Sexual Exploitation by Health Professionals, Psychotherapists and Clergy,* in Toronto, Ontario, Canada, Oct. 13, 1994.

6. John C. Gonsiorek, "Perpetrators," in *Breach of Trust: Sexual Exploitation by Health Care Professionals and Clergy*, John C. Gonsiorek, ed. (Thousand Oaks, Calif.: Sage Publications, Inc., 1995), 131.

7. Private telephone conversation with Gary R. Schoener, November 1994. An internationally acclaimed consultant on issues of professional ethics and boundaries, Schoener is a licensed clinical psychologist; a member of the faculty at the School of Public Health, University of Minnesota; a co-author of *Psychotherapists' Sexual Involvement With Clients* and *Assisting Impaired Psychologists*; executive director of the Walk-In Counseling Center in Minneapolis, Minn.; and a member of the American Psychological Association's Task Force on Sexual Impropriety.

8. From the schedule of conference events published by organizers of *It's Never O.K., The Third International Conference on Sexual Exploitation by Health Professionals, Psychotherapists and Clergy,* held in Toronto, Ontario, Canada, Oct. 13-15, 1994.

9. This description of sexual harassment is based to a great extent upon material presented in "Sexual Harassment in the Workplace: Corporate Strategies for Protection and Defense," a seminar handout (Providence, R.I.: Licht & Semonoff, Attorneys at Law, May 2, 1995).

10. Linda Greenhouse, of *The New York Times*, "Same-Sex Harassment Ruled Illegal," as the article appeared in *The Providence Journal-Bulletin*, Tuesday, March 5, 1998, A-1, 11.

11. Greenhouse, "Same-Sex Harassment Ruled Illegal," A-1.

12. Michael S. Kimmel, "Clarence, William, Iron Mike, Tailhook, Senator Packwood, Spur Posse, Magic . . . and Us," in *Transforming a Rape Culture*, Pamela R. Fletcher and Martha Roth, eds. (Minneapolis: Milkweed Editions, 1995), 130-131.

13. These five steps for preventing sexual harassment are based on the list of preventive measures presented in the seminar handout "Sexual Harassment in the Workplace: Corporate Strategies for Protection and Defense."

14. These five steps for preventing sexual misconduct are adapted from the harassment-prevention measures presented in the seminar handout "Sexual Harassment in the Workplace: Corporate Strategies for Protection and Defense."

— *6* —

How Misconduct Occurs

> One of the desert fathers, living his ascetic life many centuries ago, said that if one thinks of fornication one can avoid committing it, whereas if one fails to give sufficient consideration one invariably winds up in the wrong bed. Abba Cyrus of Alexandria was no stranger, it seems, to the dangers of allowing powerful drives to remain hidden in the unconscious mind.[1]

Sexual misconduct usually begins with a very minor violation of doctor/patient boundaries—a first step on "the slippery slope," as Linda Bowers puts it in her eponymous article about boundary issues in the doctor/patient relationship.[2] Few health-care professionals intend any impropriety. But the boundary violations that constitute sexual misconduct can begin very slowly, with apparently harmless deviations from standard procedures. A doctor may bend the rules a little bit, then a little more, until the little deviations have added up to something far from harmless.

Minor violations often set the stage for the further rationalizing of one's behavior—that is, for kidding oneself. What can a health-care practitioner do to avoid inadvertently becoming involved in such a situation? Awareness of the breakdown of professionalism is one of the major keys to avoidance.

THE BREAKDOWN OF PROFESSIONALISM

There are many ways in which the professional boundaries can fail. "Transforming the relationship to meet the [professional]'s needs is the core exploitative quality. Sex is merely one possible exploitative outcome, noteworthy because it is more noticed."[3] The following are only a few of many possible examples,[4] but when a practitioner begins to act in any of these ways, it is time for him or her to step away from that slippery slope.

Getting Too Personal. Excessive self-disclosure on the part of the doctor is a reversal of the doctor and patient roles—the patient begins to care for the care-giver. It creates an emotional intimacy that may lead to physical intimacies. "In fact, excessive self-disclosure is the single most common precursor to professional-client sex in the thousands of cases we have seen. In particular, the disclosure of current problems, especially in a significant relationship, is predictive of trouble."[5]

Making Special Financial Arrangements. The payment method breaks down. This is an indication that a doctor is beginning to think of a patient as something other than a patient. And when monetary compensation is not being provided, some professionals may begin to expect less appropriate substitutes.

Changing the Rules. Changing office policies, or your behavior regarding office policies, sets a dangerous precedent. Once the line those policies represent has been crossed—or redrawn—where does that process end?

Prolonging Treatment. Spending extra time on office visits with a particular patient, or continuing treatment for longer than the patient's condition warrants, is a sign that a doctor's attitude toward that patient is less than professional.

Neglecting Record-Keeping. This may indicate an awareness, conscious or unconscious, that there is something to hide. "There was a time when many organizations were advised by counsel to keep sparse records . . . . [But] the notion that one can retrospectively concoct a favorable version of events is quite misguided. Physicians, psychologists, social workers, clergy, and those who oversee their work do not make effective liars."[6]

TWO FLAWED MODELS OF MISCONDUCT

Let's look at two of the most commonly held beliefs about responsibility for sexual misconduct.[7] People generally believe that either the doctor is at fault or the patient is at fault.

The Rotten Apple Model

If you believe that there are some bad doctors who need weeding out, and that you have some responsibility to weed them out, then your beliefs fall into the "Rotten Apple" model of sexual misconduct. In the Rotten Apple model, there are a few sick doctors out there—they may look normal, but they can fool us—and _they_ cause all the problems. I'd like to point out some of the flaws in this model.

First, it finds no need for action beyond getting rid of the rotten apples; if doctors are either good or bad, then there is no reason to bother with training.

The second flaw is that it doesn't categorize lesser degrees of sexual misconduct as a problem—only behavior that is obviously sick—and may not take seriously anything less than forcible rape.

The third flaw is that, with this belief system, practitioners can feel very safe, believing that they could not possibly become involved in such a situation, because *they're* not sick.

The Rotten Apple is a common belief system—but if this model doesn't fit your beliefs, perhaps the next one will.

The Seductor/Seductress Model

If you believe that the patient is to blame, then you might think the source of evil is within the patient. This is like believing that women who were raped were asking for it. We'll call this "The Seductor/Seductress Model," although usually it's a woman [who is blamed]. This belief system goes back a few thousand years—to Adam and Eve! There are problems with this model, too. Let's look at some of them.

The first flaw is that, in this model, the only action called for is to protect the *doctors* from their seductive patients.

The second flaw is that, in focusing on the patient, we lose sight of the actions of the doctor, ignoring his or her abusive and damaging behavior.

The third flaw is that with this attitude, we further hurt the very people who have already been hurt.

And the fourth flaw is that, for years, this approach has very effectively silenced other victims with valid complaints. Having seen others treated as evil and as liars, who in their right mind would come forward?

The Rotten Apple and the Seductor/Seductress models both have flaws—neither fully explains who is responsible, and neither can really solve the problem of sexual misconduct. We need to look deeper, to gain a better understanding.

CULTURAL CONTRIBUTORS TO MISCONDUCT

One of the places we need to look is at our culture—at how we see the world and how we experience it. The Rotten Apple model and the Seductor/Seductress model did not arise independently, but sprang from our culture's beliefs and attitudes. There are several cultural contributors that play a role in the incidence of sexual misconduct by increasing patient or doctor vulnerability.

A Belief in Entitlement

First, there is the belief in sexual entitlement. It goes something like this: "I'm entitled to sexual relations with anyone who inspires sexual feelings in me; with anyone to whom I'm attracted; and with anyone who accepts some item or service from me." This pervasive belief system, in which sex becomes a right or a commodity, can play a major role in sexual misconduct. The patient might feel grateful or indebted to the doctor, and might see sex or sexually charged activities as a means of expressing that gratitude or discharging that debt. As a result, the patient may offer sexual favors, or may accept unwelcome advances. The doctor might rationalize that, having provided the patient with valuable, high-status services, and perhaps even the miracle of restored health, he or she is entitled to more than just money. If both the doctor and the patient are thinking this way, a volatile and potentially explosive situation is created.

A Lack of Education

Second, there is ignorance. When even doctors are unsure where they should draw the line, it is not surprising that patients also are relatively unaware of what is and is not appropriate behavior. Patients traditionally have left their common sense at the door of the doctor's office—and have been encouraged to do so. Likewise, our society teaches that doctors always act in the best interest of their patients—but it does not always teach doctors how to recognize what that is, or how to serve it.

A Deference to Power

Third, there is the power of the doctor role. Patients often not only look up to doctors because of their high social status, but also come to their doctors as penitents or petitioners. This creates at least a temporary willingness on the patient's part to go along with whatever the doctor says or does, without stopping to think it through. This phenomenon also can be observed in other relationships where the distribution of power is unequal, as between employers and employees, or men and women: "[If] women are more likely to conform to other people's ideas in social situations (a tendency noted in some research), it may be due to their typically inferior social status."[8] The usual training in politeness and the natural tendency to accede to the wishes of a higher-status individual can serve a person well in many situations, but in a situation involving coercion or abuse, they may betray him or her.

Ironically, two additional factors that may influence a patient to cooperate when a care-giver behaves inappropriately are a history of abuse and a fear of violence.

A History of Abuse

Statistics tell us that, within the United States, one in three girls and one in four or five boys have been sexually abused by the time they reach the age of eighteen. And having been abused, an individual may be more likely to submit to further abuse, in a situation where such behavior is expected.

If the abuse took place in a situation where protesting or fighting back didn't help, then the patient may have learned not to protest or fight back. Such patients may still feel utterly helpless to control their own fate. This "learned helplessness," a phenomenon observed even in animal studies, generally plays a role in keeping children with abusive parents, altar boys with abusive priests, women with abusive husbands, and patients with abusive doctors. Such a patient may feel that his or her only value, especially to a person who he or she perceives as more powerful, is as a sexual object.

A Fear of Violence

The final common factor that may increase one's vulnerability to abuse is a fear of violence. This fear is particularly common among women in our society; and again, statistics show us that they have a good reason. About 25 percent of women in the United States eventually become victims of domestic violence. Of female murder victims, about 50 percent are killed by boyfriends, husbands or ex-husbands.[9] A staggering 92.2 percent of women in our society have experienced sexual harassment, attempted rape, rape or child sexual abuse.[10]

Women are more frightened of potential violence against them than men can possibly know. Any behavior that evokes this latent fear can make them vulnerable; and out of fear, they may submit to treatment that they would never permit voluntarily. And because our culture sees power as sexy in men, and capitulation as sexy in women, the assailant may fail to realize that his victim was not seduced but simply intimidated.

A fear of violence, a past history of violence and/or abuse, a lack of certainty about what behavior is inappropriate in a doctor/patient relationship, and our culture's ideas about sex and sexuality all can contribute to the problem of patient vulnerability. The stress of illness or injury, the very thing that brings the patient to the doctor, can increase that vulnerability dramatically. Some patients are so vulnerable that they can be taken advantage of very easily.

WHO COMMITS SEXUAL MISCONDUCT?

> "Not every professional in distress is capable of sexual exploitation; rather, all professionals, when at their worst, are capable of engaging in a greater degree of boundary violation than they otherwise might imagine."[11]

Who commits these acts of misconduct? Surveys of psychiatrists indicate that they do, at the rate of about 5 to 10 percent.[12] Surveys of their patients, however, indicate that the rate may be as high as 20 percent.[13] Statistics are less available for other specialties—but psychiatrists are simply a more frequently surveyed group of health-care practitioners; there is no reason to believe that they commit misconduct any more frequently than other practitioners.

The great discrepancy between the incidence of improper behavior reported by patients and that reported by practitioners appears to indicate a high level of either denial or naïveté on the part of the offenders. This conclusion is supported by another finding: Many practitioners who report that they have engaged in behavior that meets the definition of sexual misconduct decline to describe their behavior as exploitative or harmful.

Interestingly, rather than admitting fault, the offenders often attempt to justify their behavior.

Many offenders cite a "therapeutic" intent (such as helping patients gain self-esteem or eliminate neuroses) for their inappropriate sexual behavior.   Or they may assert that their actions were appropriate but misunderstood.   If a doctor's actions are "misunderstood" in the same way by many patients, however, then the doctor is the one who has been doing the misunderstanding.

Some offenders try to justify their behavior on the basis of their own needs and desires. But these have no place in the doctor/patient relationship.

Another common justification for inappropriate or abusive behavior is love, with a majority of offenders characterizing their patients as having been in love with them when the incident occurred.

Finding a patient attractive is not an unusual phenomenon; in fact, it probably happens to the average physician on a daily or weekly basis. It is how a physician deals with this attraction that can determine the potential course toward, or away from, misconduct.

Types of Offenders

John C. Gonsiorek and Gary R. Schoener describe the following categories in their "Tentative Typology of Professional Offenders."[14]

Psychotics. These are seriously disturbed professionals—"a diverse group categorized together for convenience. They have in common impaired reality testing and significant functional impairment. They demonstrate great variability in their understanding of the effects of behavior upon victims and in their ability to feel remorse. In terms of dealing with the legal system . . . their behavior is also unpredictable."[15]   A doctor who is psychotic may believe he or she has a special connection with God; that his semen is curative; or that he or she has special powers.

"Classic" Sex Offenders.   This group includes "chronic repetitive pedophiles and also physically aggressive sex offenders regardless of the age of the victim. . . . The focus of the pedophile or the aggressive nature of the inappropriate behavior is so distinctive that we classify them separately even though there may be other dynamics operating."[16]

Impulsive Character Disorders. "Their problem behaviors are not limited to boundary violations but may include insurance fraud, sexual harassment of staff or trainees, poorly controlled sexual behavior in their personal lives, tax fraud, and a wide variety of inappropriate or criminal activity. They lack planfulness and cunning, do not cover their tracks, and so are easily caught once investigated. . . . [T]hey rarely have a true appreciation of the effects of their behavior on victims."[17]

Sociopathic/Narcissistic Character Disorders. Though also lacking impulse and behavior controls, these offenders generally are "cool, calculating, and detached and often carefully select clients who are vulnerable and/or lacking in credibility should they complain. They may be respected professionally for their skills. They are cunning enough to maintain appropriate boundaries in some situations, particularly ones in which they have public exposure. . . . and are adept at outmaneuvering others."[18]

Medically Disabled. These are professionals with good past records "who, because of a medical condition [most commonly, neurological problems or bipolar mood disorder], engage in inappropriate behavior with clients."[19] For those who have bipolar illness (also known as manic-depression) good control often can be achieved with medication.

Masochistic/Self-Defeating. "A peculiar mix of both neurotic and character disordered features. . . . [They] often appear on the surface to be overworking therapists like the more severely neurotic/socially isolated type." Except that, "because of their internal conflicts about setting limits . . . . with borderline personality or similarly disturbed patients, their otherwise reasonable clinical practice deteriorates. They become seriously impaired and boundaryless, at times with behavior involving romantic and sexual contact. It is typical in this group to find other examples of masochistic and self-defeating behavior, for example, not collecting fees, not taking adequate care of themselves . . . generally being long-suffering and self-defeating.[20]

Severely Neurotic and/or Socially Isolated. "[T]heir problems are long-standing and more significant. They often have ongoing depression, feelings of inadequacy, low self-esteem, and social isolation. Work tends to be the center of their lives and most of their personal needs are met in the work setting. Their inappropriate romantic or sexual involvement with clients . . . is repetitive in the sense that every few years, or even every decade or so, the situation re-curs. Inappropriate boundaries develop as in the healthy/neurotic group. . . [but] rooted in long-standing problems." There may be a role reversal, in which the patient starts helping the provider with his or her problems—a relationship that may easily become sexual. "They may rationalize that, because they truly love a client, the behavior is not inappropriate; because they were vulnerable or open, they had equalized the relationship; and so on. They may vacillate between self-revelation, remorse, defensiveness, and self-justification."[21]

"Simply stated, such therapists need to get a life and keep a life outside of work—but they rarely do. . . . They are often regarded among other profes-sionals as particularly giving, skilled, dedicated, and hardworking professionals. . . . However, the same factors that predispose them to this dedicated behavior also predispose them to periodic, repetitive, severe boundary violations with a small number of their clients.[22]

Naïve. These practitioners may be unaware of personal or professional boundaries, "Some . . . may simply not know (or may have such simplistic understandings that they might as well not know) about sexual impropriety with patients." They may "not literally believe it is permissible to have sex with a patient. [But] typically, they are naïve about ethical gray areas that, once trans-gressed, often eventuate in increasingly inappropriate and boundaryless behavior that may result in sexual misconduct. They are naïve about the trajectory of their behavior and start down the 'slippery slope.' "[23]

Normal and/or Mildly Neurotic. "These individuals potentially constitute all health care professionals and clergy.'' Under severe stress, such as the loss of a spouse or a significant relationship, people become vulnerable and impulsive. In such a state, it is possible for a very sudden, intense emotional connection to occur.

Typical "is a reasonably well-trained, responsible professional who, at a bad spot in his or her life [and is] socially isolated, depressed, and lacking in adequate support . . . . A client who fits his or her countertransference like lock and key enters the caseload. The professional begins a slow and gradual process of developing a romantic attachment to the client, often by inappropriate self-disclosure, moving to social interaction, and sometimes . . . proceeding to romantic and sexual interaction. Such individuals literally fall in love with their patients. . . . Almost without exception, these perpetrators have one and only one victim.''[24]

"It is our impression that the number of these perpetrators is not small. It is one of the most common groups that we have assessed [at the Walk-In Counseling Center].''[25]

An Alternative Categorization

Glenn O. Gabbard of the Nenninger Clinic, to whom Gonsiorek gives credit for recognizing the Masochistic/Self-Defeating offenders as a separate category, is among the researchers who group offenders somewhat differently. Here are his categorizations:

> The vast majority of therapists who become sexually involved with patients will fall into one of the following four groups: (a) psychotic disorders, (b) predatory psychopathy and paraphilias, (c) lovesickness, and (d) masochistic surrender.
>
> The first category, psychotic disorders, is definitely the smallest group of the four and consists of therapists who suffer from such disorders as bipolar affective disorder, paranoid psychoses, schizophrenia, and psychotic organic brain syndromes. They generally require extensive treatment that includes pharmacotherapy and vocational counseling [that is, steering them into another career].[26]

WHO IS AFFECTED BY SEXUAL MISCONDUCT?

> Sexual abuse of all kinds represents a gross failure in the empathic concern one person has for the subjective experience of the other.
> —*Judith V. Jordan,*
> *"The Movement of Mutuality and Power,'' 1991*

Many doctors rationalize that their intimacies with their patients were beneficial or neutral experiences for the patients; they may justify the episode either on the basis of their own needs and concerns or by citing the supposed benefit to the patient.[27]

It should be noted, however, that "psychiatrists who later treated such patients reported that the sexual contact was harmful to the patients.''[28] And in Canada, the Ontario College of Physicians and Surgeons sponsored one of the largest studies to date of the problem of non-psychiatric sexual misconduct. The study concluded that these violations of trust in the physician/patient relationship were ''devastating''—for the patient, for the patient's family, for the public's trust in the health-care professions and for our society as a whole.[29]

Effects on Doctors

Loss of Reputation. The doctor's reputation may be negatively affected, if accusations become public.

Loss of Income. The doctor's practice is likely to suffer as news or rumors about a sexual offense drive away patients, and it will be further damaged if the doctor loses time from the practice to hearings or a trial.

Loss of Relationships. The doctor's relationships with others are likely to be hurt, whether by the sense of accusations themselves, or by the stress of legal proceedings. Divorce and other break-ups are not uncommon.

Loss of Assets. Because many malpractice insurance policies do not cover incidents of misconduct,[30] the doctor may lose large amounts of money to attorneys' fees, even if no judgement is entered against him or her.

Loss of Livelihood. The doctor's license might be suspended or revoked.

Loss of Freedom. The doctor might face possible imprisonment.

Effects on Colleagues

Other doctors in the area could also suffer loss of reputation and of income, especially if media coverage is involved. For some of them, this might lead to problems with relationships.

Effects on Professions

In a high-profile case, the profession of the accused doctor, and related professions, are likely to lose both trust and prestige.

Effects on Patients/Victims

The marks that sexual misconduct leaves on its victims are many. (For further discussion of the aftereffects of sexual abuse, see Chapter 7, ''Caring for The Abused Patient.'') These are just a few of the most common:[31]

Loss of Identity. Having been treated as an object, a victim may feel that he or she really is nothing more than an object.

Loss of Self-Esteem. The victim may feel used; unclean; good only for sex; unworthy of normal courtesy and a healthy relationship.

Depression. The victim may suffer from mild to severe clinical depression, and may even become suicidal.

Post-Traumatic Stress Syndrome. The victim may suffer physical and emotional exhaustion, and may be so profoundly affected that he or she has trouble functioning; *housekeeping, finances, and relationships* all may suffer.

Guilt/Self-Blame. The victim may feel he or she was somehow at fault. Such feelings, often encouraged by the perpetrator, are a major contributor to depression.

Isolation. The victim may feel cut off from all sources of support—especially if he or she is keeping the abuser's secret.

Loss of Boundaries. The victim may have difficulty reestablishing the boundaries that have been violated. This lack of firm boundaries makes him or her even more vulnerable to subsequent sexual misconduct or abuse.

Loss of Health Care. Once the relationship with the abuser ceases to be entirely professional, the care the victim receives is likely to suffer. Later, a lingering distrust of doctors may pose a continuing barrier to appropriate care.

Two Examples of Sexual Misconduct

Here are the real-life stories of two patients who became victims of sexual misconduct; they illustrate many of the points already discussed. The names have been changed to protect the privacy of all concerned.

Deborah Roe. Deborah Roe became a patient of Dr. Smith's because she was experiencing health problems that were within his area of expertise; he had been highly recommended.

Within several visits of her initial appointment, she began to like and trust him. He became friendlier and friendlier as time went on. He opened up to her and shared more and more personal information about himself. This made her feel special and liked. In time, he began to call her on the phone to tell her what was happening in his life. Their time together in the office started to include long hugs, and more touching of a friendly nature began to take place.

They never progressed to sexual intercourse, but there was significant sexual misconduct. None of this happened overnight—it was a gradual process. The patient remarked that there had been numerous times along the way when their relationship could have gone back to strictly doctor/patient, but the doctor did not take the opportunity to steer in it in that direction.

Once, after the contact between them had progressed to kissing and fondling, she recalls having told him that perhaps she should be seeing another doctor. He said: "I can handle it!" At that point, Deborah says, she figured, "he's the doctor and he knows what he's doing." She did not realize that, not only was their behavior contrary to her best interest, since she had come to him for care and her care was suffering, but also that it was illegal for him to be kissing her in the office.

Deborah's life was thrown into a frenzy as a result of the relationship, particularly when she discovered that other women had also had such experiences with Dr. Smith. This discovery shattered the belief in him that she had tried to preserve. She felt used, betrayed, and devalued as a person—and isolated, because he had not wanted her to tell anyone. Her spirit was harmed.

She finally went to the licensing board and filed a formal complaint. The doctor did not lose his license, but he did forfeit his reputation and much of his practice.

Deborah had previously been sexually abused by a health professional. When she was 19, her fiance had died in an automobile accident. Naturally distraught, she had sought the help of a counselor at the college she was attending. The counselor provoked her into a sexual relationship that also involved drugs. He had her believing that she was crazy and that she needed drugs. It turned out that the drugs he had given to her required supervision because they were so dangerous—and he was not supervising their use. Her experience with this counselor helped to set the stage for future abuse by a health professional or anyone else in a power position.

John Doe. John Doe was fit, handsome and charming, and that was half the problem. He also had a very strong sex drive, but did not find masturbation to be satisfying, and his wife had little interest in sex. So when women became interested in him, which was often, he generally followed up on that interest.

At any one time, he would have a handful of willing female friends and acquaintances whom he used for sexual gratification. He did not form serious relationships with these women.

Eventually, as his marriage was falling apart, John came to recognize that his approach to sexuality was unhealthy; he sought out a psychologist to help him learn to deal with his compulsive behavior. The doctor he was seeing—the woman who was supposed to be helping him to reduce his reliance on casual sex—entered into a sexual relationship with him.

Ironically, the very pattern that he was trying to break by seeking therapy was duplicated and reinforced by the professional to whom he turned for help. John's psychotherapist told him that she found him very attractive. She said she felt that she could no longer do her job, since this attraction was interfering.

After just a few sexual incidents, John realized that this new relationship was making his situation worse. He says that he questioned his own value. His feelings didn't seem to count, even with someone whom he was paying to address those feelings. He says he felt like a sex object. His personal pain was ignored and increased, so that the psychotherapist could gratify her own desires.

He describes the entire experience as a setback. But, he says, he feels fortunate that he was an older patient who could more easily weather the emotional storm that overtook him during and after the affair with his psychotherapist.

He is now seeing another psychotherapist.

COMMON FEARS AND MISCONCEPTIONS

> I would urge women and men to appreciate the deep but differing fears the phenomenon referred to as "sexual harassment" engenders in the other.
> Men should try to understand women's abiding fear of male violence and their reluctance to offend by stating that something makes them uncomfortable.

This, I think, is what lies behind the familiar refrain that some men "just don't get it."

But women, for their part, should try to understand men's fears of being falsely accused, of having a woman they felt protective toward turn on them and destroy them.

—*Deborah Tannen,*
"Talking from 9 to 5," 1994

Just as sexual harassment generates fears in both men and women, so sexual misconduct engenders fears in both doctors and patients. Some of these fears have a basis in fact, some do not. Here are some of the most common fears and misconceptions.

Doctors' Fears
The "Fatal Attraction." A common fear is that an angry, rebuffed patient will stalk or torment the doctor. A perhaps less improbable scenario is that the doctor will be haunted by an angry abuse survivor who feels that he or she was denied justice.

The Temptress. Many doctors fear an irresistible patient, who will somehow lure the doctor into doing wrong. But anyone who has so little control of his or her sexual impulses that this is a realistic possibility should not be working in a health-care profession.

False Complaints. Many doctors fear that they will be falsely accused, but very few false complaints are filed. Through the late 1970s, there were very few complaints of any kind, and those that were filed received short shrift. In the last two decades, the social cost of filing a complaint against a physician has decreased, while the likelihood that such a complaint will be taken seriously has increased. This has been followed by an increase in complaints, as had previously been seen with rape and sexual harassment cases; at some point—as has already been seen with rape cases—these improvements in the complaint process are likely to bring an increase in false complaints.

False Censure or Conviction. While not impossible, this is highly unlikely, at least in the current regulatory atmosphere. In an analysis of hundreds of cases of physicians, clergy, and psychotherapists who had been censured or convicted for sexual misconduct, the Walk-In Counseling Center in Minneapolis, Minn., found not a single instance in which the decision was not fully supported by the facts.[32]

An Innocent Mistake or Misunderstanding. For doctors who lack training in touch, sexuality and boundary issues—that is, for most doctors—this is a serious risk. They may unknowingly violate laws and boundaries by acting in ways that are improper or unsafe.

Patients' Fears
The Vengeful Perpetrator. Patients fear that, if they complain, their abuser

will come after them. While this has been known to happen, it is far from likely, although the doctor and his or her legal team may attack the patient's reputation.

Disbelief. Victims fear that they will not be believed, or that their complaints will not be taken seriously.

Blaming the Victim. They fear that even if they hated and objected to what happened, even if they struggled to prevent it, they may be accused of "asking for it."

Self-Blame. Some victims of sexual misconduct are afraid that—having consented to what happened, or having failed to object strenuously enough to prevent it—they might be to blame. Like victims of other forms of sexual abuse, they are likely to suffer from feelings of shame and self-loathing.

Inaction. Patients fear that filing a complaint will do no good; that even if they complain and are believed, no action will be taken. Often, they have been correct.

A Living Nightmare

Probably the most common fears among victims of sexual misconduct are that they will not believed, or that, even if they are believed, the perpetrator will not be published. Both of these fears came true for psychiatric patient Barbara Nöel, whose book *You Must Be Dreaming* chronicles her own real-life experience of sexual misconduct.

For seventeen years, Nöel had been seeing an internationally renowned psychiatrist—Jules Masserman, a former president of the American Psychiatric Association—who drugged her at many sessions with sodium amytal, an addictive and dangerous barbiturate. He told her that these "amytal interviews" were necessary, to permit them to explore issues that her conscious mind was not ready to address. Finally, during one of these "interviews," she came to a little early. She awoke to discover that her psychiatrist was having sexual intercourse with her. "After Dr. Masserman blinked the light on and off, I'd usually lie there for another half hour, but not this time. Not when I knew what he had done to me. Not when the repulsive stench of his body odor and the after-shave lotion wafted up from my own shoulders and made me feel like gagging."[33] The odors were familiar; for years, she had thought they were a side-effect of the drug. Now she knew better.

After leaving her psychiatrist's office, she went straight to the office of another doctor in the same building. After she decided that she wanted to report the rape, she was referred to a hospital for examination. There, she was questioned by the police—by a male officer who ridiculed her story and tried to get her to say that she had imagined the whole experience:

> "Now, wouldn't it be better to assume you might have been dreaming all this?"
> "No," she said. "I was *not* dreaming."
> ". . . You're saying that you couldn't have been dreaming this?"

"I was *not* dreaming this," she said.

"But you could have been, couldn't you, ma'am?"

"Yes, I suppose I *could have been*, but I wasn't."

"I felt like shouting at him," she said later. "Did he think a woman would go to the hospital—get herself wheeled in to be poked and prodded and disbelieved and totally humiliated, with people asking insulting and irrelevant questions . . . and not even allowed to pee—just to have a little fun with these guys or waste their time?"[34]

After this initial experience, it took years—and lawsuits from four other women, who also had been patients of Jules Masserman—before Barbara Nöel saw any results. In 1987, Masserman consented to give up his license to practice medicine or prescribe drugs in Illinois. In 1991, he was suspended for five years from the American Psychiatric Association and from the Illinois Psychiatric Society. But as of 1992, when Nöel's book was published, he continued to serve on the American Psychiatric Association's Board of Trustees.

NOTES

1. Susan Howatch, *Absolute Truths* (New York: Fawcett Crest, 1994), 323.

2. Dr. Linda J. Bowers, "Back to basics . . . The 'Slippery Slope': Boundary Issues for the Chiropractic Physician," *Topics in Clinical Chiropractic* 1 (1994) 3, 1-8.

3. John C. Gonsiorek, "Assessment for Rehabilitation of Exploitative Health Care Professionals and Clergy," in *Breach of Trust: Sexual Exploitation by Health Care Professionals and Clergy*, John C. Gonsiorek, ed. (Thousand Oaks, Calif.: Sage Publications, Inc., 1995), 149.

4. The first three examples are based upon comments by Gary R. Schoener, M.A., and John C. Gonsiorek, Ph.D., in their workshop "Assessment, Treatment and Supervision of the Professional Offender," presented at *It's NEVER O.K., The Third International Conference on Sexual Exploitation by Health Professionals, Psychotherapists and Clergy*, in Toronto, Ontario, Canada, Oct. 13, 1994.

5. Gary R. Schoener, "Employer/Supervisor Liability and Risk Management: An Administrator's View," In *Breach of Trust: Sexual Exploitation by Health Care Professionals and Clergy*, John C. Gonsiorek, ed. (Thousand Oaks, Calif.: Sage Publications, Inc., 1995), 308.

6. Schoener, "Employer/Supervisor Liability and Risk Management," 305.

7. The following section is adapted from the transcript of the keynote address by Dr. Angelica Redleaf, "Beneath the Surface: A Deeper Look at Sexual Misconduct," that was delivered at the 62nd Annual Congress of the Federation of Chiropractic Licensing Boards, in Portland, Ore., on May 11, 1995 (Warwick, R.I.: Association for Chiropractic Excellence, Inc., 1995).

8. Diane E. Papalia and Sally Wendkos Olds, *Psychology*, 2nd ed. (New York: McGraw-Hill Book Company, 1985), 426.

9. Patricia Aburdene and John Naisbitt, *Megatrends for Women* (New York: Villard Books, 1992), 282.

10. Gail E. Robinson, Rachel Edney, Joan Bishop, and Stella Blackshaw, "Preventing Sexual Exploitation in Doctor-Patient Relationships through Medical

Training," A conference session presented at *It's Never O.K., The Third International Conference on Sexual Exploitation by Health Professionals, Psychotherapists and Clergy.* Toronto, Ontario, Canada, Oct. 14, 1994.

11. John C. Gonsiorek, "Assessment for Rehabilitation of Exploitative Health Care Professionals and Clergy," in *Breach of Trust: Sexual Exploitation by Health Care Professionals and Clergy*, John C. Gonsiorek, ed. (Thousand Oaks, Calif.: Sage Publications, Inc., 1995), 149.

12. Howard Brody, *The Healer's Power* (New Haven, Conn.: Yale University Press, 1992), 22.

13. Linda Mabus Jorgenson, "Sexual Contact in Fiduciary Relationships: Legal Perspectives," in *Breach of Trust: Sexual Exploitation by Health Care Professionals and Clergy*, John C. Gonsiorek, ed. (Thousand Oaks, Calif.: Sage Publications, Inc., 1995), 237.

14. Gonsiorek, "Assessment for Rehabilitation of Exploitative Health Care Professionals and Clergy," 147-154.

Gary R. Schoener and Gonsiorek also discussed their "Tentative Typology of Professional Offenders" in their workshop "Assessment, Treatment and Supervision of the Professional Offender," presented at *It's NEVER O.K., The Third International Conference on Sexual Exploitation by Health Professionals, Psychotherapists and Clergy,* in Toronto, Ontario, Canada, Oct. 13, 1994.

15. Gonsiorek, "Assessment for Rehabilitation of Exploitative Health Care Professionals and Clergy," 152.

16. Gonsiorek, "Assessment for Rehabilitation of Exploitative Health Care Professionals and Clergy," 152.

17. Gonsiorek, "Assessment for Rehabilitation of Exploitative Health Care Professionals and Clergy," 150-151.

18. Gonsiorek, "Assessment for Rehabilitation of Exploitative Health Care Professionals and Clergy," 151.

19. Gonsiorek, "Assessment for Rehabilitation of Exploitative Health Care Professionals and Clergy," 152-153.

20. Gonsiorek, "Assessment for Rehabilitation of Exploitative Health Care Professionals and Clergy," 153-154.

21. Gonsiorek, "Assessment for Rehabilitation of Exploitative Health Care Professionals and Clergy," 149-150.

22. Gonsiorek, "Assessment for Rehabilitation of Exploitative Health Care Professionals and Clergy," 150.

23. Gonsiorek, "Assessment for Rehabilitation of Exploitative Health Care Professionals and Clergy," 147-148.

24. Gonsiorek, "Assessment for Rehabilitation of Exploitative Health Care Professionals and Clergy," 148.

25. Gonsiorek, "Assessment for Rehabilitation of Exploitative Health Care Professionals and Clergy," 148.

26. Glen O. Gabbard, "Psychotherapists Who Transgress Sexual Boundaries With Patients," in *Breach of Trust: Sexual Exploitation by Health Care Professionals and Clergy*, John C. Gonsiorek, ed. (Thousand Oaks, Calif.: Sage Publications, Inc., 1995), 135.

27. Nanette K. Gartrell, Nancy Milliken, William H. Goodson III, Sue Thiemann, and Bernard Lo, "Physician-Patient Sexual Contact: Prevalence and Problems," in

Breach of Trust: Sexual Exploitation by Health Care Professionals and Clergy, John C. Gonsiorek, ed. (Thousand Oaks, Calif.: Sage Publications, Inc., 1995), 21.

28. Gartrell, Milliken, Goodson, Thiemann, and Lo, "Physician-Patient Sexual Contact: Prevalence and Problems," 19.

29. Gartrell, Milliken, Goodson, Thiemann, and Lo, "Physician-Patient Sexual Contact: Prevalence and Problems," 25.

30. Even those insurers who do not provide sexual misconduct coverage may be named in misconduct suits against their malpractice-insurance clients, and may therefore be saddled with substantial attorney's fees. Several insurance companies, therefore, have decided to educate their policyholders about misconduct, in hopes of minimizing the number of such problems that will arise in the future.

One example is the handbook, by Michael J. Stahl and Stephen M. Foreman, entitled *Sexual Misconduct: Ethical, Clinical and Legal Ramifications for the Chiropractic Profession* (Des Moines, Iowa: NCMIC Insurance Co., 1997).

31. These examples of effects exhibited by victims of physician sexual abuse are based in part upon the comments of Robinson, Edney, Bishop, and Blackshaw, in "Preventing Sexual Exploitation in Doctor-Patient Relationships through Medical Training," a conference session they presented at *It's NEVER O.K., The Third International Conference on Sexual Exploitation by Health Professionals, Psychotherapists and Clergy*, Toronto, Ontario, Canada, on Oct. 14, 1994.

Also helpful was the work of Gartrell, Milliken, Goodson, Thiemann, and Lo, in "Physician-Patient Sexual Contact: Prevalence and Problems," 18-28.

32. Telephone conversation with Gary R. Schoener, M.A., November 1994.

33. Barbara Noël, with Kathryn Watterson, *You Must be Dreaming* (New York: Poseidon Press, 1992), 120.

34. Noël, with Watterson, *You Must be Dreaming*, 126.

— *7* —

Caring for the Abused Patient

Sexual abuse is an all-too-common phenomenon. The greatest of care must be exercised, therefore, in caring for all patients, because any one of them may be a survivor of rape, violence, or abuse. Remember the First Law of Medicine: "First, do no harm."

Patients who previously have been abused need to be treated with particular sensitivity and care, not only because they have been traumatized but also because, having once been abused, they have become more vulnerable to further abuse. "When a person has been abused and violated by caretakers . . . all relationships become infused with distorted sexual and aggressive elements."[1] Someone who has suffered abuse may have been left with a feeling of utter helplessness that makes it impossible to resist coercion; may have been led to believe that he or she is worthless except as a sexual plaything; or may have learned to think of sex as a currency with which to purchase affection and approval.

At least one in four Americans have been abused by the time they reach the age of eighteen. Thus, whether they know it or not, all doctors probably are caring for a significant number of patients who have been sexually abused. Chances are, however, that a doctor won't know which patients they are. Abuse survivors rarely identify themselves.

A SURVIVOR'S TALE

I heard a speaker—at a conference I attended in Toronto, in Ontario, Canada—who talked about his own experience of sexual abuse.

He is a Cree Indian, from northern Canada. When he was a child, it was common for the government to remove Indian children from their families when they were about six years old. And this is what happened to him: He was sent to a Catholic residential school. Naturally, there were priests there. These priests went around to each child's bed after the lights went out and proceeded to masturbate the children nightly. Imagine the terror. You're six years old. Away from your family. It's dark. And the priest is *on* you. What scars would that leave? And what would your experience be like in a doctor's office after that?

Will we know which patients *have been* abused, sexually or otherwise? Do you know how to care for such patients? They *need* special care.[2]

Because so many people have been abused, all office procedures, behavior, and communication should take these large numbers of potential abuse survivors into account. And because statistics indicate that the overwhelming majority of those who abuse children are men, the care of abuse survivors is particularly problematic for male practitioners. The former victims generally will be the most vulnerable and the most anxious or fearful in the presence of those who most resemble their former abusers.[3]

SIGNS AND SYMPTOMS OF ABUSE

People who have been abused, sexually or otherwise, may suffer from post-traumatic stress syndrome, which combines both psychological and physiological symptoms. These symptoms could include anxiety, fears, extreme startle responses, and intense reactions to stimuli associated with the traumatic event. Abuse survivors also may have sleep disorders or suffer from depression.

These symptoms are so common that they are of only limited usefulness in identifying abuse survivors. If confronted with such symptoms, however, it is helpful to be aware that abuse may be their cause. Patients exhibiting such behavior need special care, whatever the cause of their condition.

STAGES OF RECOVERY

Three stages are commonly described in the recovery from sexual abuse: safety, reconstruction and reconnection. But it should be noted that abuse survivors do not necessarily recover in a neat, linear manner. There often is much moving back and forth from one stage of recovery to another. And for many patients, the process will never be complete.

1. *Safety:* The traumatized individual starts to regain control of his or her life and needs, such as nutrition, sleeping, exercise, and a safe place to live.

2. *Reconstruction:* Reliving or reconstructing the traumatic experience. Once the victim feels safe, memories may begin to resurface.

3. *Reconnection:* The former victim begins to rebuild his or her life and regain the ability to trust others.

GUIDELINES FOR THE PRACTITIONER

Potential Pitfalls

When you know that a patient has been abused, there are several very important points to keep in mind:

Don't Fall into the "Rescuer" Trap. Do not try to take on the entire burden of the patient's healing by yourself. The rescuer fantasy of believing you and you alone have the power and the gift to save someone can be very attractive, and very dangerous. A patient's perceived need for rescue and a practitioner's perceived ability to provide it have been the basis for the rationalization of all kinds of boundary infractions, including sexual misconduct. Such "white knight" aspirations are among the most narcissistic and dangerous of traps.

Don't Get in Over Your Head. Caring for a patient who has not yet reached the third stage of recovery can present problems that most practitioners are unprepared to handle.

Don't Work Without a Net. When working with a patient who has been severely traumatized, especially if he or she is still in the early stages of recovery, be certain that the patient has a safety net—a psychotherapist, and a network of friends—so that you do not become the sole source of support.

Don't Get Burned. Patients who have been abused may feel that their only value is as a sex object; some may encourage, request, or even demand a sexual relationship. Be prepared to deal with this possibility. Caring for such patients can be like juggling with fire, and should not be attempted without adequate training and support.

Proper Preparation

If you wish to care for patients who have been sexually abused, study the field of sexual abuse—read the literature, take the classes, and learn from the experts.

Consider Entering Psychotherapy. Working with a therapist or counselor can be helpful in exploring your own attitudes toward power and sexuality, in teaching you about the therapy experience your abused patients are likely to be going through, and in helping you to cope with the stresses and challenges that are likely to arise in treating such patients.

Consult the Patient's Psychotherapist. If a patient is in counseling or psychotherapy and also needs intensive care from you, let him or her know that you would like to discuss the case with the psychotherapist. If the patient agrees, get a written authorization from the patient and then speak with the psychotherapist. Ask relevant questions, such as: Is this patient ready for body work? Are there specific guidelines that should be offered in caring for this patient? What sorts of problems are most likely to arise in providing this patient with physical care? Is there any area of the body that should be avoided?

Stay in Touch. Ask the patient's psychotherapist whether the lines of communication between you can be kept open. Ask to be informed of any new issues that arise in the course of the patient's counseling that might be relevant to the care that you provide.

Treating the Abuse Survivor

After getting the go-ahead from the psychotherapist to work with this patient, you'll still need to abide by some very basic rules:[4]

Set Goals Together With the Patient. Involve him or her in any decision that will affect his or her care. This will help to prevent misunderstandings, and also may help to restore the patient's sense of autonomy.

Empower the Patient. Educate him or her about the rights and power of patients and individuals; encourage the patient to exercise these rights.

Build Emotional Safety. Show respect for the patient as an individual. Show compassion for his or her experience. Never do anything without his or her consent.

Be Prepared for Flashbacks. Memories and emotions may be triggered as the patient is touched. Like scent, touch is a powerful trigger for memory.

Be Deliberate. Remain aware of the pace of touch, and be meticulous about obtaining consent for every procedure, for every touch. Keep things sedate and predictable; avoid surprises.

NOTES

1. Nancy A. Bridges, "Meaning and Management of Attraction: Neglected Areas of Psychotherapy Training and Practice," *Psychotherapy*, 31 (Fall 1994): 3, p. 431.

2. The autobiographical account of sexual abuse of young Cree Indian children was told by noted Canadian playwright Thomson Highway in his plenary address, "It's Never O.K.: A Personal Viewpoint," at *It's Never O.K., The Third International Conference on Sexual Exploitation by Health Professionals, Psychotherapists and Clergy*, Toronto, Ontario, Canada, Oct. 15, 1994.

This retelling of Mr. Highway's story is taken from the transcript of Dr. Angelica Redleaf's keynote address, "Beneath the Surface: A Deeper Look at Sexual Misconduct," presented at the 62nd Annual Congress of the Federation of Chiropractic Licensing Boards, in Portland, Ore., May 11, 1995 (Warwick, R.I.: Association for Chiropractic Excellence, Inc., 1995).

3. From the transcript of Dr. Angelica Redleaf's keynote address, "Beneath the Surface: A Deeper Look at Sexual Misconduct," presented at the 62nd Annual Congress of the Federation of Chiropractic Licensing Boards, Portland, Ore., May 11, 1995 (Warwick, R.I.: Association for Chiropractic Excellence, Inc., 1995).

4. For sources of more detailed information on treating patients who are survivors of physical or sexual abuse, see Suggested Reading, at the back of this book.

— 8 —

Boundaries and Consent

PERSONAL BOUNDARIES

We've mentioned boundaries before; now, let's consider them more thoroughly. People often refer to the interests or activities they share with someone else as their "common ground." Fritz Perls, the father of Gestalt Therapy, calls this place where two people meet the "Mitwelt." This is a German term that means the middle world or middle land. It's the place where two people have a connection, where their lives come together.

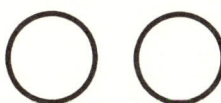

Strangers:
People with no Mitwelt

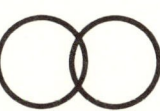

Acquaintances:
People with a small Mitwelt

The first of these diagrams represents two people who do not have any relationship—they are strangers. The second represents two people who have a relationship, who interact with each other on their common ground. Because we are people, not circles, each of our lives may overlap with someone else's in several areas. But—apart from certain special relationships, such as that of a parent with a young child—each person should remain an intact, distinct personality. They interact, they overlap, but they do not blend or merge.

The closer two people are, and the younger they are, the more blending and merging—the more crossing or blurring of boundaries—are likely to take place.

In a relationship where there is an imbalance of age or of power, the older or more powerful individual has an obligation to look out for the welfare and protect the boundaries of the person who is younger or less powerful.

Boundaries also can imagined as being "like a cell wall—a semipermeable membrane letting some things in, and keeping others out."[1]

PROFESSIONAL BOUNDARIES

A professional boundary combines social, psychological, and physical components. Some limits are established by law; some, by ethics; some, by professional associations; some, by the individual. A professional boundary differs from a personal boundary in that, as a professional, a person is held to a higher standard than a nonprofessional. Implicit in the professional relationship is a legal obligation, on the part of the professional, to put aside personal needs and wants, in order to better serve and respect the needs and wants of the person being served.

When we enter into a professional relationship with another person, our personal as well as our professional boundaries need to be kept very distinct. That is easily said, but not always so easily accomplished. Some people have fragile boundaries that are easily shattered; some people have fuzzy boundaries that are easily blurred. And even a person who usually has well-defined boundaries may become vulnerable during a period of stress.

Duties of the Professional
The doctor and patient need to be careful of and for one another, to avoid violating either personal or professional boundaries. The professional must:

- respect the patient's physical and psychological personal space;
- respect the patient's beliefs;
- respect the patient's body;
- ensure proper and appropriate two-way communication;
- deal with the patient nonjudgmentally;
- take care not to harm or exploit the patient;
- do what is proper and ethical and best for the patient.

If all is going well with the patient, then the doctor can relax and pay a little less attention to policing the boundaries, but he or she still needs to be very aware of patient behavior and communication. The doctor must remain alert to any sign that the boundaries need to be tightened up again.

Responsibilities of the Patient
The clients in a professional relationship also have the opportunity to prevent boundary violations. In order to protect themselves, patients should:

- ensure that their personal space is respected;
- demand that their beliefs be respected;
- demand that their bodies be respected;
- work to ensure proper and appropriate communication;
- guard against exploitation;
- demand that they be cared for properly and ethically.

Patients also should be extremely aware of everything that happens in the interaction with the care-givers and the office staff. If all is going well, the patient can then ease up on the wariness, but should continue to watch for shifts in the doctor's or staff's behaviors or attitudes.

Mutual Watchfulness; Mutual Protection
It behooves patients to be watchful of their care-givers because, as has become more and more clear, professionals are fallible humans, like everyone else; they cannot be given *carte blanche*.

It likewise behooves health-care practitioners to be watchful of their patients. It is neither safe nor appropriate to assume that all patients will be guarding and protecting themselves, or will even be capable of doing so. Those patients who do not or cannot protect themselves should be treated with special care and concern. Just as the power is the professional's in the doctor/patient relationship, so is the responsibility.

Why Boundaries Matter
When both doctor and patient are concerned about one another's boundaries, then both doctor *and* patient are protected. Yet, even though they have always been important, the boundaries between the patient and the professional are an issue that only recently achieved prominence.

Problems may arise when a doctor has remained unaware of professional boundaries. He or she may unknowingly cross the line—and, in the process, may unknowingly harm patients. But *lack of awareness is no excuse*. Doctors still are responsible for conducting themselves in the manner that their professional status requires.

Problems also may arise when a doctor's personal boundaries are weak. If the patient's personal boundaries are weak, as well, then problems may be compounded, or may escalate out of control.

Any time that patients are hurt, the health profession that is represented also is hurt. Recall how the profession of psychiatry has suffered, following the media coverage of scandalous behavior by psychiatrists. When, for whatever reason, the professional boundaries between doctor and patient are not respected and maintained, then everyone loses: the patient, the doctor, and the profession all suffer perhaps irreparable harm. The only winners—if any—are the attorneys who profit from the lawsuits.

Only when health-care professionals fully understand their role, their power, their personal biases and concerns, and the impact of all relevant factors on the doctor/patient relationship is it possible to be reasonably sure that the professional boundaries that protect us all will be honored and respected.

THE QUESTION OF CONSENT

Sexual Consent

Many people believe that, where sexual involvement has occurred between a doctor and a patient, the patient was "asking for it" and really wanted it. This is the Seductor/Seductress Model of sexual misconduct. We could go on and on with arguments to counter such a belief—but perhaps the strongest is simply this: *Legally and ethically, it doesn't hold water.*

The courts have ruled that patients are not in a position to give consent for sexual or romantic involvement. Notable examples include a case heard in 1975 before the New York State Second District Court (*Roy v. Hartogs*), between a psychiatrist and his patient, which cited the psychiatrist's "position of overwhelming influence and trust"; and a case heard before the Supreme Court of Canada in 1992 (*Norberg v. Winrib*), concerning a doctor who supplied a patient with painkilling drugs in exchange for sex.[2] The decision in this latter case noted that:

> Patients seek the help of doctors when they are in a vulnerable state—when they are sick, when they are needy, when they are uncertain about what needs to be done. . . . The unequal distribution of power in the physician-patient relationship makes opportunities for sexual exploitation more possible than in other relationships. This vulnerability gives physicians the power to exact sexual compliance. Physical force or weapons are not necessary because the physician's power comes from having the knowledge and being trusted by patients.[3]

Because a patient's vulnerability may give doctors the power to exact sexual compliance, the health professions also have taken a dim view of doctor/patient sexual involvement. "The patient/doctor relationship must be one of absolute confidence and trust," the Australian Medical Association declares. "Patients and their families must be confident that doctors will not take advantage of the professional relationship to indulge in sexual behavior of any kind. Seeking to shift the blame from the doctor to the patient is not acceptable."[4]

The American Medical Association ruled in 1989 that physician/patient sexual activity is not ethical, if it takes place while the professional relationship is in force. And the American Chiropractic Association, in presenting the advisory opinion of the ACA Ethics Committee that having "sexual intimacies with a patient is unprofessional and unethical," urges its physicians to "do nothing to 'exploit the trust and dependency of the patient.' "[5]

Procedural Consent

The importance of obtaining the patient's full, informed consent for every procedure and every touch cannot be over-stressed. Touching a patient without consent is more than unwise. It also is rude, presumptuous, unduly intimate, and perhaps illegal. Even treatments or diagnostic procedures that are clinically appropriate can be traumatic—and problematic—if they are not understood or if they are imposed upon an unwilling patient. When consent is given short shrift by health-care professionals, as too often is the case, several issues arise:

Informed Consent. Since the Kennedy administration, in the early 1960s, the full, informed consent of the patient or the patient's guardian has been a prerequisite for most patient care—except in certain emergency situations involving a patient who is for some reason not capable of giving such consent.[6]

The patient has the right to withhold consent, or to withdraw consent at any time. Even if given, the patient's consent is not considered to be valid unless the patient has been informed about the procedure itself, the reason for performing the procedure, and the risks and possible benefits, and also has been informed about any reasonable alternatives to the procedure. What is more, the explanations must have been comprehensible to the patient and must actually have been understood by the patient.

Assault. In many jurisdictions, though the law is seldom so strictly interpreted, any uninvited touch can be held to constitute assault. Exceptions often are made for accidental touch, depending to some extent on the circumstances. Bumping into or brushing against another passenger on a crowded bus, for instance, would tend to be looked upon more leniently than coming into similar contact with someone in an uncrowded hallway.

Sexual Misconduct. Even diagnostic or therapeutic procedures that are clinically appropriate may constitute misconduct under some circumstances. To take an extreme example, consider the situation of an uninformed patient subjected to an examination of the breasts or testicles: He or she is gowned or draped when someone rushes in, uncovers a very private portion of the patient's anatomy, stares at it, gropes it, and leaves. Even finding out later that the someone was a doctor, the staring was a visual examination, the groping was palpation for abnormal masses, and the procedure was a screening for cancer would not erase the trauma that the patient had already experienced.

NOTES

1. Larry A. Spicer, from the outline for his address "Professional Boundaries for the Federation of Chiropractic Licensing Boards," which was delivered at the 62nd Annual Congress of the Federation of Chiropractic Licensing Boards, in Portland, Ore., in May 1995 (Minnesota: Larry A. Spicer, April 1996), 2.

2. Linda Mabus Jorgenson, "Sexual Contact in Fiduciary Relationships: Legal Perspectives," in *Breach of Trust: Sexual Exploitation by Health Care Professionals and Clergy*, John C. Gonsiorek, ed. (Thousand Oaks, Calif.: Sage Publications, Inc., 1995), 241.

3. Jorgenson, "Sexual Contact in Fiduciary Relationships," 241-242.

4. Australian Medical Association, "Sexual Conduct Between Doctors and Their Patients: Position Statement—October 1994," as posted on the association's World Wide Web page, Australian Medical Association Limited, 1995.

5. "Addendum: Sexual Intimacies with a Patient," the ACA Code of Ethics, 1994-1995 (American Chiropractic Association, 1994), 10.

6. Examples of conditions that may render a patient incapable of giving full, informed consent include youth, mental illness, intoxication or other disorientation, and unconsciousness. (Hence, the importance of "living wills" to people who wish that certain procedures *not* be performed, should they become incapacitated.) In cases where a patient is partially impaired, however, it generally is considered that procedures should be explained and consent obtained to such an extent as the patient's condition permits.

— *9* —

The Doctor Role

The word "role" had its origins in the theater; it began to find its way into the literature of the behavioral sciences as early as the 1920s. The roles we take on in life are learned, just as actors in the theater must learn the roles that they play. And each role that we experience—for example that of mother, father, teacher, friend, patient, doctor—is fraught with cultural meaning and steeped in tradition. The doctor's role is particularly complex and intriguing.

THE POWER OF THE DOCTOR ROLE

The role of the health-care practitioner is imbued with a symbolism far more powerful than that of any individual in our society. The doctor role traditionally is active, whereas the patient role is passive. The doctor role is powerful, while the patient role traditionally is powerless. The doctor role is very knowledgeable, while the patient role traditionally is not.

These roles, once learned, are difficult to change. "One reason lies in the unconscious nature of this kind of social interaction. Like speaking a well-rehearsed part or driving a car, the many words and actions that make up 'acting like a doctor' and 'acting like a patient' become automatic and escape our awareness." Another factor is a "mortal fear of committing improprieties" that inspires people to work hard at maintaining their social roles, regardless of whether to do so is in their best interests.[1]

When doctors begin their education, they are not yet comfortable in the traditional doctor role. Many start out being familiar with only the role of patient. But, slowly, they are indoctrinated into the mysteries of the doctor's role, and they are granted the symbols of their new power.

Let's go back to when you first started feeling the power of this role:

Remember when you purchased your *first* white clinic jacket and your *black bag*? Wasn't it an awesome feeling?

That was around the time when we were initiated into our power as healers. Over time, we became comfortable with our power. As time passed, our power became invisible—to us. But it is never invisible to our patients. That's the power of our role.

We need to remember that power, and the profound effect it has on our patients—we need to remember it so we don't misuse it.[2]

PARTNERSHIP AND POWER

> [I]f one shares the power precisely with the person in greatest danger of
> being victimized, the potential for self-correction of error seems greatest.
> —*Howard Brody, M.D.,*
> *"The Healer's Power," 1992*

Power, which is an integral part of the doctor/patient relationship, as it is in any relationship, requires a certain vigilance so that it is not abused. There is good reason to be watchful for signs of power becoming imbalanced: The greater the imbalance, the greater the potential for abuse.

The traditional doctor/patient relationship is hierarchical; that is, most of the power rests with the doctor. A number of methods have evolved for reinforcing this hierarchy. These include the use of the above-mentioned white coat and black bag, as well as many methods that are not so benign. Often, the doctor's power is hoarded rather than shared; it is gained at the patient's expense.

For instance, doctors may insist on the use of professional titles for themselves and their staff. This is fine—unless, as is commonly the case, patients are not accorded the same courtesy. Then it becomes a matter not of respect, which is a two-way street, but of condescension. Similarly, patients are expected to be show up on time for their doctor's appointments. Yet at many offices, they are routinely kept waiting. "This has come to be one of those institutionalized rudenesses of the profession," writes the modern-day etiquette expert who is known as Miss Manners.[3] This expectation of promptness and patience also has come to be one of the chief complaints patients have about doctors.

Even worse, what is sacrificed in this process may be not the patient's dignity, but doctor/patient communication. This is an outcome that is particularly unfortunate giving the quelling effect that is already exerted on doctor/patient communication by the very power imbalance these tactics are designed to exaggerate. (Further discussion of doctor/patient communication is presented in Chapter 1, in The Effect of Doctor Gender, on pages 23-25; and in this chapter, in Power and Communication, on page 101.)

For instance, patients seldom are permitted to finish describing a complaint or answering a question before they are cut off. This costs the doctor information that might have been invaluable in arriving at a diagnosis, or in deciding what treatment options to pursue, and is likely to leave the patient feeling irritated, frustrated, flustered, or intimidated—not the ideal state of mind for answering questions or accepting advice. Likewise, the doctor's advice may be dispensed quickly and with little explanation, but with much technical jargon. The effect is impressive, yet indecipherable—especially if questions are discouraged.

In the partnership model of health care, by contrast, respect and accommodation are mutual. But the partnership is not, it should be noted, entirely an equal one. The doctor still has the advantage of superior skills and knowledge; the patient still has the vulnerabilities that may be created by the very illness or injury for which he or she seeks treatment.

This more-equitable model also is more popular with patients—and it may well prove a more effective variant of the health-care relationship. Studies have shown that, when patients have a greater degree of equality with their doctor, they fare better. Their health has also been seen to improve proportionally to their participation in doctors' visits; more talking, more asking of questions, and a more assertive patient role all seem to contribute to this phenomenon.

There are many indicators that female doctors tend to prefer and be more comfortable in a partnership with their patients. There also are many indicators that this role has, to a great extent, been forced upon them. Our society is not very accepting of women who embrace the traditional male style of leadership.

Three Kinds of Power

In his book *The Healer's Power*, Howard Brody describes three distinct kinds of power in the doctor/patient relationship:[4]

1. *Aesculapian Power.* This form of power is based on the physician having knowledge. This knowledge is imparted through professional training, and encompasses knowledge about the body, medicines, therapies, drugs, and so forth. Anyone with sufficient intelligence—and time—can learn these things.

2. *Charismatic Power.* This form of power is based on the degree of charm possessed by the individual practitioner. A physician either has charisma or lacks it. To a great extent, it can't be learned.

3. *Social Power.* This form of power is based on the status that society gives to a particular health profession. This can change from generation to generation, from time to time, and from place to place, with shifts in the society.

Three Patterns of Power

Another way in which power can be classified is in cooperative terms—rather than hierarchical terms—on the basis of how it affects and is affected by our relationships with others.

1. *Power Over.* Whenever we gain power, we also gain the possibility of using it to control others.

2. *Power With.* When we share our power *with* others, we use it for their benefit as well as for our own.

3. *Power From.* Examples are our professional title and our position. We also may gain power from professional or personal associations with others, or from being related to, knowing, or working for someone important. But when we have gained power from a source outside ourselves, it is easier to take for granted. How careful are we likely to be with it?

Our society's culture of the Independent Man particularly values "power over"—power over oneself, power over others, power over nature—and it is this kind of power that has become an integral part of the health-care relationship. Differences between male and female practitioners in this area have been well-documented, particularly the contrast between the male tendency focus on control and hierarchy and the female tendency to focus on concern and connection.

Uses of Power

The final consideration is how power is used; that is, where the power is directed. Is it used to control others? Is it shared with others? Do we take advantage of the power of our role? Do we abuse our power? Brody lists three ways that power can ethically be used in the health-care relationship:[5]

1. *Owned Power.* Those who have power can acknowledge that they have it.

2. *Shared Power.* Those who have power can give some of it up to their patients, or can direct it to the benefit of those they care for.

3. *Aimed Power.* Those who know that they have power must be aware of how and at whom they're aiming it.

Until recently, the power held by health-care professionals was not even acknowledged. But now, this long-unspoken power is in the process of shifting away from its exclusive resting place in the hands of health professionals, and toward the hands of the patients. "Today's patients are more knowledgeable and insistent on sharing crucial decisions. Today's doctors are slowly changing to meet their demands."[6] One of the areas in which this change has been manifested is in changing attitudes toward the concept of patient compliance.

ADHERENCE vs. COMPLIANCE

As we (slowly) move away from the paternalistic conception of the doctor-patient relationship, to a form of the relationship where the patient's autonomy and fundamental right to self-determination is acknowledged, we should also abandon the present conception of compliance. If it is ultimately the patient who has to decide, after being duly informed and advised, then he cannot be non-compliant. He may be non-collaborative, obstructive, foolish or stupid if he blatantly disregards the decisions to which he is a party, but since they *are* decisions and not the doctor's orders, this does not imply non-compliance.

—Søren Holm, M.A.,
"What Is Wrong With Compliance?" 1993

Compliance

In the compliance model of health care, the patient is given orders by the doctor. These orders may or may not be explained, but the patient is expected to follow them to the letter. Patients who ask too many questions or who decide not to do what is expected of them are "noncompliant" or "bad."

Adherence

In the adherence model, the patient is informed about his or her condition. The doctor then suggests options for care, which are explained to and discussed with the patient. But it is the patient who makes the final decision. Patients are advised to adhere to the agreed-upon course of treatment, but are never expected to give up their right to decide what they want for themselves.

There are a number of reasons why doctors are cautious about giving up some of their power and allowing the patient to take on more of it. A doctor has a lot riding on whether the patient follows through with his or her recommendations. There is the patient's well-being; there is the risk of a malpractice suit; and there are the doctor's ego and reputation—all of which add to the complexity of the changing doctor/patient relationship.

It turns out, however, that adherence may be a better way of achieving the patient follow-through than the old model of forcing compliance upon patients. Compliance studies show that few patients actually follow their doctor's orders. Consider this analysis of a survey by *Consumer Reports*:

> [A] disturbing number of our readers with chronic disorders aren't taking the drugs they need. Strict adherence to drug therapy is essential for people with diabetes, arthritis, or elevated blood-cholesterol levels. Yet more than one in four people with those problems said they didn't follow doctor's orders. But, if they felt their doctor cared, they were more likely to follow through with recommendations.[7]

POWER AND COMMUNICATION

An excellent example of the power of roles affect communication is presented by Deborah Tannen, in *Talking from 9 to 5*, when she describes a conversation that was recorded between the pilot and co-pilot of a commercial airplane shortly before a fatal crash: "The co-pilot knew that something was wrong, but he was unable to directly tell the pilot, the authority figure . . . . The co-pilot repeatedly called the pilot's attention to dangerous conditions but did not directly suggest that they abort the takeoff."[8]

Unfortunately, the pilot did not correctly interpret the co-pilot's hints. The results of this miscommunication were tragic. In a subsequent analysis of numerous flight-crew conversations, Tannen reports that "it was typical for the speech of subordinates to be more mitigated."[9]

A person of lower status tends to have more difficulty speaking up in the presence of a person of higher status. This is every bit as true in a doctor's office as it is in the cockpit of an airplane; and in a doctor's office, as in an airplane, the results of miscommunication can be tragic. Yet, like the supremacy of pilot over co-pilot, the superior status of the doctor over the patient traditionally has been maximized. It is vital that the power of our role be understood, so that we can care for patients optimally: with respect, awareness, and integrity.

Both patients and doctors are affected by their respective roles, in ways that are both conscious and unconscious. The names that are given to this effect are transference and countertransference.

TRANSFERENCE AND COUNTERTRANSFERENCE

We've learned that patients rarely see their health-care provider as just another human, with his or her own set of frailties and problems, with whom they can comfortably speak about anything. It's much more common for patients to see their doctor as any one or some combination of the following: all-knowing, indifferent, above the mundane everyday concerns of the rest of humanity, rich, perfect, cold, all-caring, the answer to all of their prayers, or someone not to be trusted. Much of this is so because of the power of our role.

Transference
In order to understand the power of the role of doctor more completely, it is useful to look to the fields of psychology and psychiatry for their contribution in this area. Trainees in the fields of psychology and psychiatry learn that clients/patients frequently develop a role transference toward their health-care providers. In other words, a patient unconsciously transfers to the care-provider the feelings, attitudes, and behaviors from his or her relationship with one or more individuals in the patient's past. This transference often takes the form of the patient seeing the provider in something akin to a parental role; in his or her relationship with this provider, the patient may feel or behave more like a child than an adult.

When handled with care and awareness in counseling and psychiatry, transference makes it easier to work through issues from the patient's past relationships. In a health-care relationship where there is no knowledge of this process, however, practitioners can run into unforeseen difficulties. Transference, when it affects the patient, naturally has tremendous consequences for the doctor.

Countertransference
We've seen that transference complicates the doctor/patient relationship. But there is another, similar process called countertransference, which involves the doctor transferring his or her feelings or behaviors to the patient. What happens in a countertransference situation is that the doctor begins to feel toward the client the same way that the doctor felt toward someone in his or her past. This phenomenon may involve wanting or even needing to rescue the patient, or feeling a particularly close bond because of a similar life experience. In

either case, it is not the current relationship that is bringing out these feelings but a similar dynamic from the past.

Under the influence of such doctor/patient connections, both doctor and patient may do and say things that they would not ordinarily. This makes it very important for all health professionals to understand the effects of transference and countertransference.

Traumatic Transference and Countertransference

Patients who are suffering from a traumatic syndrome often develop a particular type of transference in a therapy or a health-care relationship. Their prior traumatic experience has severely distorted their responses to anyone in a position of authority. Because of their feelings of helplessness at the time of the abuse, they often feel abandoned. Clearly, knowledge of such bondings between a traumatized patient and his or her care-giver can be a valuable tool in caring for those who have been abused.

There are a number of ways in which we can minimize the profound effect of the doctor role on both doctor and patient. Among these are sharing our power with patients; sharing our knowledge; sharing *appropriate* aspects of ourselves; and watching for signs of transference and countertransference, both in ourselves and in our patients.

NOTES

1. Debra L. Roter and Judith A. Hall, *Doctors Talking With Patients/Patients Talking With Doctors: Improving Communication in Medical Visits* (Westport, Conn.: Auburn House, 1992), 17.

2. Angelica Redleaf, from the transcript of the keynote address, "Beneath the Surface: A Deeper Look at Sexual Misconduct," delivered at the 62nd Annual Congress of the Federation of Chiropractic Licensing Boards, in Portland, Ore., May 11, 1995 (Warwick, R.I.: Association for Chiropractic Excellence, Inc., 1995), 6.

3. Miss Manners (syndicated columnist Judith Martin), "Sick of Doctors Testing Patience in Waiting Room," *The Providence Sunday Journal*, Feb. 26, 1995, H-6.

4. Howard Brody, *The Healer's Power* (New Haven, Conn.: Yale University Press, 1992), 16.

5. Brody, *The Healer's Power*, 43.

6. Joan Cassell, *Expected Miracles: Surgeons at Work* (Philadelphia: Temple University Press, 1991), 151.

7. "How Is Your Doctor Treating You?" *Consumer Reports*, 60 (February 1995): 87-88.

8. Deborah Tannen, *Talking from 9 to 5: How Women's and Men's Conversational Styles Affect Who Gets Heard, Who Gets Credit, and What Gets Done at Work* (New York: William Morrow and Company, 1994), 93.

9. Tannen, *Talking from 9 to 5*, 94.

— *10* —

What Is the Solution?

THE FAILURE OF SELF-REGULATION

History tells us that physician sexual misconduct is nothing new. It is a problem that at a minimum is nearly as old as the history of medicine, and that probably is as old as medicine itself. There are few historical references to misconduct itself, but many to society's attempts to solve it—generally, by self-regulation of the health-care professions, with ethical codes and credos indistinguishable from those in use today.

> [E]thics codes, discussion, and research alone have failed to significantly change the situation. We have tried "Plan A"—self-regulation in concert with codes of ethics—and it has not solved the problem. Twenty-four centuries is probably long enough to try any one solution. Now it is time for new initiatives.[1]

People and governments around the world are beginning to take steps toward developing new solutions to the problem of sexual misconduct. Canada has taken many.

EXTERNAL REGULATION

Ontario Province
In Canada, the province of Ontario took a major step toward new initiatives with a massive study in the late 1980s and early 1990s. The purpose of the study was to determine just what the extent of the problem of sexual misconduct is in Ontario, as well as to better define the problem itself. A task force was appointed, and its findings were published. As a result of this study, some major steps were taken by the Ministry of Health in Ontario. This project is

extremely complex, as are the actions in which it has resulted, so we'll take just a brief look at some of what has been done. Ontario has:

- created very strong legislation barring sexual misconduct by health-care providers;
- instituted mandatory training for health-care professionals;
- instituted mandatory reporting of abuse by colleagues;
- created protections for patients who come forward;
- agreed to provide therapy for those who have been abused.

The Ontario Task Force on Sexual Abuse of Patients recommended a tiered definition of sexual misconduct, dividing offenses into two categories: sexual impropriety and sexual violation.

Sexual Impropriety. This is the lesser category of offense; very briefly, it may include some of the following:

a. Any behavior, gesture, or communication that is seductive or sexually demeaning to a patient. Examples include flirting; comments about body or clothing; calling people by terms such as honey, sweetie, cutie, bitch, whore, stud, fox, or bastard; or using inappropriate words to describe body parts.

b. Making comments about the patient's potential sexual performance, or requesting details about the patient's sexual history and preferences, except when and as clinically indicated.

c. Telling the patient about the practitioner's sexual problems, preferences, history, performance, or fantasies.

d. Inappropriate procedures, such as failing to gown patients when they are asked to disrobe, or examining or touching a patient's genitals without a glove.

e. Asking a patient for a date.

f. Kissing a patient.

Sexual Violation. This is the more serious category of sexual misconduct offense, for which the study panel recommended a minimum penalty of a five-year suspension from practice. It consists of engaging with a patient in any conduct that is sexual, or that may reasonably be interpreted as sexual. The panel cited a number of behaviors that would qualify, including the following:

a. Performing examinations of the breasts, the genitals or the rectal area that are not clinically appropriate; for which the patient has not given consent; or for which the patient has withdrawn consent.

b. Engaging in physician/patient sexual intercourse, or other physician/patient sexual acts, whether initiated by the patient or the physician.

c. Masturbating in the patient's presence, or encouraging the patient to masturbate in the physician's presence.

No miraculous change has been seen in Ontario since the study panel's recommendations, in revised form, were adopted into law. Implementation of the law and of the other measures has sometimes been neither swift nor smooth. But as Melissa Roberts-Henry, a former victim of abuse by a therapist, wrote of the 1988 Colorado law criminalizing sexual contact between psychotherapists and their patients:

Several difficulties remain despite the law's existence. These include poor treatment of victims/survivors during the investigation process or unwillingness of prosecutors to proceed with cases due to lack of understanding of abuse. Nonetheless, *the law is a significant achievement.* For, while the law may not work perfectly or be of benefit in each individual case, there have been and will continue to be benefits from the statute that accrue to society as a whole: increased public awareness, making perpetrators responsible for their actions, and, in the ideal situation, removal of abusers from the mainstream where it is likely that they will continue to do harm.[2]

Around the World

Steps similar to those taken in Ontario also have been taken in other provinces of Canada, and in other parts of the world, such as in England and Australia—but they are needed elsewhere.

Without similar actions on the part of the health professions and the government agencies that regulate them, more patients will be harmed; and more doctors, many of whom simply have no idea that their behavior could be harmful, also will suffer. All health-care professions will feel the consequences of inaction.

PROFESSIONAL MONITORING

In psychology and psychiatry, clinicians are guided throughout their careers by ongoing supervision from a trained supervisor, to help them maintain clear boundaries between clinician and patient/client. Such assistance would be a tremendous asset in other health-care fields, as well.

The mental health fields have long recognized the impact of role on the helper/helpee relationship and, particularly, the influence of transference and countertransference. That is part of the reason these professions so strongly recommend ongoing supervision from an experienced counselor for all their practitioners. Such external monitoring is viewed as essential to maintaining an ethical practice.

Supervision can be provided one-on-one or in a group setting (see page 122). Either way, such a meeting is an opportunity for the doctor to discuss situations and feelings that arise as part of caring for patients. A group setting "broadens the base of learning and creates an additional support system for each member. . . . Hearing the fears and doubts of other practitioners who are feeling challenged by unusual client situations can help one to feel less isolated and alone."[3]

When it has been integrated into the physical health-care professions as well, supervision can be expected to bring heightened awareness of the complexity of the roles of doctor and patient and heightened safety for both parties in the doctor/patient relationship.

EDUCATION AND INDIVIDUAL SELF-MONITORING

Meanwhile, what is a doctor to do? Actually, a great deal—and, if you are reading this, you're already on your way. There are many actions that practitioners can take to help prevent problems with sexual misconduct. These include learning more about what behavior is acceptable; evaluating your current level of risk; gaining better communication skills; and adapting office practices to minimize risk and discomfort. Part III, the Patient Protection Protocol, focuses on steps that individual doctors, practices, and other health-care organizations can take to help create greater safety and satisfaction for both doctor and patient.

NOTES

1. Gary R. Schoener, "Historical Overview," in *Breach of Trust: Sexual Exploitation by Health Care Professionals and Clergy*, John C. Gonsiorek, ed. (Thousand Oaks, Calif.: Sage Publications, Inc., 1995), 16-17.

2. Melissa Roberts-Henry, "Criminalization in Colorado: Overview and Opinion," in *Breach of Trust: Sexual Exploitation by Health Care Professionals and Clergy,* John C. Gonsiorek, ed. (Thousand Oaks, Calif.: Sage Publications, Inc., 1995), 347. Roberts-Henry is a survivor of sexual abuse by a psychotherapist; her story and subsequent civil court case were the subject of the PBS documentary "My Doctor, My Lover." She has gone on to found the advocacy group In Motion—People Abused in Counselling and Therapy (IMPACT), to be appointed by the governor to the Colorado State Board of Psychologist Examiners, and to co-author the state's Civil Court Rape Shield Bill.

3. Ben Benjamin, Ph.D., *Massage and Bodywork with Survivors of Abuse* (Medford, Mass.: Ben Benjamin, 1994), 73.

PART III

Patient Protection Protocol

I swear by Apollo the physician and by Aesculapius to keep the following oath: I will prescribe for the good of my patients and never do harm to anyone. In every house where I come, I will enter for the good of my patients, keeping myself far from all intentional ill-doing and all seduction, and especially from the pleasures of love with women or men, be they free or slaves.

—From the Hippocratic Oath,
in use since the fourth or fifth century B.C.

WHY "PATIENT PROTECTION"?

It is no accident that this program is called the "Patient Protection Protocol"* rather than "Practice Protection Protocol" or "Practitioner Protection Protocol." When we focus on protecting ourselves against our patients, the result is a garrison mentality. The doctor/patient relationship becomes an adversarial one: It's us against them.

When we take this stance, every patient is seen as a potential enemy, and both care and communication can suffer. Yet effective communication and good doctor/patient rapport are considered to be the best way to prevent malpractice and misconduct allegations. Although communication problems certainly are not the immediate cause of most malpractice suits, they are generally thought to be the primary predisposing factor. We believe that the same holds true for claims of sexual misconduct. What occurs within the office, and the relationships that result, may help to determine not only the level of care a patient receives but also the nature of the patient's reaction if there are problems in care later on. So it is likely that a "Practitioner Protection Protocol"—one that focused on protecting the doctor, rather than the patient—would be ineffective. Such an adversarial approach might even *increase* the frequency of patient complaints.

It is far more effective to protect a practice by protecting the patient, because it is the patient's experience of the practitioner and the practice that has the potential for creating problems. The Patient Protection Protocol helps doctors to reduce the level of risk involved in caring for our patients, by minimizing the possibility that we will allow harm to come to them.

This is not a quick fix. We'd all love to have some quick formula to minimize the problem of sexual misconduct—but such a hope is unrealistic. There *are* some immediate steps that can be taken to minimize this challenge to our practices, but to achieve true patient and doctor protection, many facets of the practice will need to be assessed. Great attention is needed to the handling of sexuality, gender, touch and power, and the way that affects patient care. The Patient Protection Protocol (PPP) includes:

Safe Touch Protocol: a system for touching patients safely and communicating with them about touch, featuring the Anatomical Risk Levels and the Safe Touch Guidelines.

Safe Practice Strategies: a guide to creating a safe and comfortable environment for patients, doctors, and staff.

Safe Practice Analysis: a method of assessing practice safety and diagnosing problems that make the practice vulnerable. It includes both the Sexual Misconduct Risk Factor Analysis (RFA), for a quick self-assessment, and the Practice Analysis Questionnaires, for an in-depth evaluation.

Making Changes: additional hints on how to classify and how to address whatever problems may have been identified by the Safe Practice Analysis.

---

* Patient Protection Protocol, Safe Touch Protocol, Safe Touch Guidelines, Safe Practice Strategies, and Safe Practice Analysis are trademarks of SafeCare, Inc.

— *11* —

Safe Touch Protocol

The Safe Touch Protocol includes both a discussion of Anatomical Risk Levels and the Safe Touch Guidelines.

ANATOMICAL RISK LEVELS

These anatomical risk levels are general guidelines, only. Any touch, at any place on the body, may have the potential to be a high-risk contact, depending on the patient's personal experience.

Risk Level I: Back, neck, face, head, hands, arms, shoulders, legs, feet.

Risk Level II: Thighs, buttocks, pelvis, hip, chest, upper abdomen.

Risk Level III: Lower abdomen, breasts, genitals, anal area, areas close to these.

How to use the Anatomical Risk Levels:

1. The first time that you care for a patient, whether at Level I, II, or III, be sure to ask for and receive permission before proceeding with touch.

2. Whenever dealing with a new patient, or a new part of a patient's body, be alert for unusual responses to touch. For instance, some patients might be very ticklish—but only in certain areas, such as the rib-cage. Other patients might have an erotic reaction to touching of a part of the body, such as the neck, that is not generally considered an erogenous zone. They might be unusually tender in some places, so that a normal firm touch causes them pain. Or they might experience disturbing memories or emotions when certain places are touched or certain types of touch are used; this is especially true of the many patients who previously have been raped or otherwise abused.

3. A patient who has previously experienced abuse that involved a particular part

of the body—the face, for example—may require special care and consent when that part of the body is touched. Or, such a patient may require special care whenever he or she is touched, anywhere on the body.

4. Each and every time you are about to touch a patient, it is vital to be alert to that patient's body language and tone of voice so that you can be certain that you have the go-ahead to proceed with touch.

5. If you know that a patient has been sexually abused, then each time you see that patient, be sure to ask for permission for each touch.

SAFE TOUCH GUIDELINES

Step I: The Pre-Touch Thinking Process

Before touching any patient—especially if that touching will involve Anatomical Risk Level II or III—the practitioner needs to go through an extensive thinking process. Initially, this process may slow things down a little; but once it has become part of your "doctoring" routine, it will take only a second or two. This process involves asking yourself the following questions:

1. Does this procedure need to be done?
2. Am I the right person to perform this procedure? Would someone else be able to do it better?
3. Do I have the ability and the facilities to ensure safety for this patient?
4. What are my motives for wanting to do this procedure?
5. Am I interested in doing this for my benefit, or for the patient's benefit?
6. If this patient was someone else, to whom I was not attracted, would I be as eager to perform this procedure?
7. Will I be putting this patient into a physically or emotionally vulnerable position in the process of performing this procedure?
8. If I will be making the patient vulnerable, am I justified in doing so?
9. Will this patient feel safe during the procedure?
10. How will I know whether the patient is feeling safe or unsafe?

When you have answered all of these questions, and you feel certain, first, that your only motivation is the best interest of the patient, and second, that the patient will feel safe, then move on to Step II.

Step II: The Pre-Touch Communication Process

Communication is essential when practitioners are about to touch a patient. We must use a communication process that is patient-centered: Our tone and our words must be clear and respectful. Explanations must be in English, not "medicalese." In other words, with the words we use, with the way we use them, and with the tone in which we deliver them, we need to show respect for the patient. With that in mind, here is how to proceed:

1. Explain to the patient why you are considering performing the procedure.

2. Tell the patient all the pros and cons of performing the procedure. Give all the information, not just the facts that build a better case for patient compliance.
3. Have charts, diagrams, and so forth available to help illustrate the need for performing the procedure and explain what you will be doing.
4. Pay close attention to the patient's reactions and questions.
5. Ask the patient what would make him or her feel safe during the procedure. If the patient doesn't know, suggest some options: having a third person present; keeping the door open; videotaping; audio taping; none of the above. Let the patient know that nothing will be done until you are certain that he or she will feel safe.
6. Explain how you will provide safety and a comfortable atmosphere for the patient.
7. Ask for the patient's consent to perform the procedure.
8. If consent is not given, do not use tactics that will make the patient feel bad. Respect the patient and his or her decision.

This process should precede touch at any of the three Anatomical Risk Levels; but when a procedure will involve a Level III contact, the process should be completed with especial care. Don't take it personally if the patient asks that someone else be in the room, or if he or she wants the door to remain open—or asks anything else, for that matter. Most likely, he or she would feel the need for the same reassurance with any practitioner.

When all communication has been completed to the satisfaction of both practitioner and patient, move on to Step III.

Step III: Providing Safety During the Procedure

Before beginning, ask yourself whether a patient who has been sexually abused and who is close to terror at the thought of being touched would feel comfortable—or at least safe—with you during the procedure. The keys are:

Respect: An atmosphere of respect is essential. Imagine that this person is an esteemed individual.

Time: Do not take longer than is necessary. Use a minimum of communication *during* the procedure; try to cover all the bases before you begin.

Touch: Use a minimum of touch. Remain aware of both hands. Take care to avoid accidental or unintended touching, especially of high-risk areas.

Practice: Take the time to practice doing all procedures, with these guidelines in mind, before caring for another patient.

Step IV: Post-Touch Communication

This is a time when the patient and doctor should discuss how the procedure went, what worked and what did not work, and what was learned. To begin:

1. Let the patient know that you appreciate his or her trust in you.

2. Tell the patient what you found. If full results from a diagnostic procedure are not yet available, then explain the reason for the delay, and tell the patient when the results will be in.

3. If you suspect a problem that will require further checking into, inform the patient of who, what, when, where, how, and why.

4. Tell the patient what benefits you anticipate from having performed the procedure.

5. Ask the patient if he or she has any questions or comments about the procedure, or about the results.

6. Discuss further diagnostic and treatment options with the patient. If there is any chance that the patient has not understood you, try asking him or her to repeat what you have said.

This post-procedural communication is important for several reasons: It helps to reassure the patient that there was a valid reason for the procedure. It may elicit valuable diagnostic data missed by the procedure itself—for instance, you may have been trying to locate tender spots, while the patient was trying to be stoic and not show pain. And if the procedure is one that will be repeated, this discussion will help both you and the patient to determine how best to proceed next time.

Step V: Post-Touch Self-Evaluation
Don't skip this valuable step; it can enlighten you about yourself and your sensitivity to patients. Ask yourself:

1. How did I do?

2. Was I respectful? Was I sensitive to the patient's wants, needs, vulnerability?

3. If a colleague or the patient's significant other or parent had been watching, would I have felt good about how I performed this procedure? About how I cared for and communicated with this patient?

4. Is there a need for any improvements, the next time such a procedure will be performed?

5. Grade yourself. For instance, if you and the patient both felt good about the way the procedure went, give yourself an "A."

If any portion of the Post-Touch Self-Evaluation indicates a need for improvement, consider getting an outside opinion about your procedures. Possibilities include peer supervision, individual or group supervision, and training.

Likewise, if the risk-assessment questionnaires in the Safe Practice Analysis (Chapter 13) highlight some behavior or attitude problems, *do* take steps to ensure your patients' safety and your own. Although it can be difficult to endure having one's behavior critiqued, it also can be very valuable. Assumptions are dangerous; instead of assuming, it can be very important to actually *know* what effect our behavior has on our patients.

Safe Practice Strategies

The Safe Practice Strategies involve paying attention to office policies and procedures, patient needs, and doctor and staff attitudes and behaviors. By so doing, we can learn what action steps are needed to safeguard our patients, our practice and ourselves.*

There are three major categories of Safe Practice Strategies: office-centered interventions, patient-centered interventions, and doctor-centered interventions. These interventions not only provide safety, but also facilitate the creation and maintenance of a successful practice. As Franklin D. Roosevelt put it, ''If you treat people right they will treat you right—ninety percent of the time.'' When patients feel are treated with care and respect, they notice—and send others.

The information that follows is only a beginning, however. No cookbook approach, however extensive, will contain the remedy for every situation that may arise in actual practice. As you make discoveries in your practice, please share them with us; your electronic visits are welcome on the Internet, at the World Wide Web site www.safecare.org. Adapting the way in which we care for patients, so that we become able to provide appropriate care to anyone who comes to us, requires a deeper assessment of ourselves, a dedication to learning, and a sensitivity to patient needs.

OFFICE-CENTERED INTERVENTIONS

These are environmental interventions; that is, they involve taking stock of the environment within the office. Office-centered interventions can be

---

* I would like to thank my colleague, Dr. Gwenneth Rae of the University of Rhode Island, for inspiring this chapter.   *—Angelica Redleaf, D.C.*

implemented immediately. Two key points to keep in mind:

- Always respect the patient's privacy and vulnerability.
- Whenever possible, give the patient the option of choosing environmental changes.

Educating Patients About Safe Practice

Posting a "Patients' Bill of Rights" in your waiting area or providing a "Patients' Rights" pamphlet to all new patients will signal to your patients that you are concerned about them. Some practitioners fear that such materials might encourage patients to complain, but they can actually be a valuable tool for preventing problems by improving communication. If a patient believes that your practice is patient-centered, then if something that you or your staff says or does makes him or her uncomfortable, the patient will be more likely to mention it you—rather than to a lawyer.

Protecting Patient Privacy

Keep Private Procedures Private. Place equipment that may be used by semi-clothed patients, such as a scale, in a private spot with private access—not in a busy hallway.

Maintain Confidentiality. Do not discuss patients or their treatment in areas where others might overhear.

Create a Changing Area. Provide a safe and comfortable place for patients to change. If no closed-door exam room exists, or if such space is at a premium, create a separate changing area to provide privacy. A door or a curtain that will stay closed until the patient is ready is vital. Provide a stable chair or bench; several sturdy hooks, or some other spot to put clothing and a purse; and a mirror, so patients can check their hair and attire before they leave. Make sure there is enough room to change comfortably, even if assistance is required.

Reducing Intimacy

Keep Exam Room Doors Open. Or, eliminate walls or doors between exam areas. This can reduce the sense of forced intimacy that results from being closeted together with another person in a small room with what is essentially a small bed. But it also can reduce or eliminate patient privacy. An open-door or open-office policy works best in situations—for instance, an outpatient physical therapy practice—where the patients remain fully clothed and their conditions are not the sort about which people tend to be embarrassed.

Have an Assistant in the Room During the Exam or Procedure. While this is often recommended as a preventive measure, it does have significant drawbacks—aside from the obvious one of cost. First, it reduces patient privacy. Second, it has the potential to impair communication, because it alters the doctor/patient dynamic; it may leave the patient feeling outnumbered. And third, it may create a false sense of invulnerability. In venues where an assistant's presence is required, this measure has not eliminated either all complaints or all actual misconduct. In the case of a doctor/patient misunderstanding or doctor misbehavior, the doctor's paid staff member will generally side with the doctor.

An assistant in the room may be essential, however, with particular patients or during particular procedures that make patients particularly vulnerable. And in some jurisdictions and some institutions, the presence of a third person is required during all procedures that require the patient to disrobe. To minimize potential adverse effects when this method is used, be sure to introduce the assistant to the patient, and remember that, when the patient is outnumbered, it may be necessary to work harder at drawing him or her out.

PATIENT-CENTERED INTERVENTIONS

Patient-centered interventions include behavioral and procedural interventions, and involve assessing the safety and comfort of patients during all procedures. They also include assessing the level of risk to the patient in all procedures. In other words, they involve the doctor and staff putting themselves in the patient's shoes.

These interventions can have some real, long-lasting effects; they also could take some time to fully implement. Implementing each specific procedure or technique requires that thought be given to whether all patients will be comfortable and feel safe. Some general guidelines to keep in mind:

- The more disrobing, the greater the risk.
- The more touching, the greater the risk.
- The more isolated the doctor and the patient are, the greater the risk.

Obviously, the greatest risk is encountered when there is a high-touch procedure, little clothing, and doctor and patient are alone.

Remember, this list is only a beginning. As you make discoveries in your practice, make those changes that you deem necessary.

Disrobing, Gowning and Draping of Patients
Depending upon your type of practice, disrobing, gowning, and draping might be an everyday, if not an every-patient, requirement. This may already be handled perfectly and respectfully in your practice; however, please take the time to consider these details. You may discover points that you had not considered.[1]

Selecting Gowns. Choose gowns that are thick enough and large enough to actually provide good coverage. Get the opinions of people you trust regarding the selection of gowns. Be prepared to provide two gowns, if necessary, to patients of greater girth.

Instructing Patients. Give patients clear instructions about your office's gowning procedures. Tell them what clothing they should remove. Tell them what they should put on, where it is, and how it should be worn. After the exam or treatment is completed, be sure to let patients know when they can put their own clothing back on.

Establishing Readiness. Establish a system that patients can use so that people won't walk in while they are changing. This system could be to have everyone knock and ask "Are you ready?" before opening the door to an exam room. It could be to have the patient open the door a crack, or flip a switch to turn on a signal light outside the door. It could be some other way of letting the doctor and staff know that the patient has changed and is ready.

Providing Assistance. Unless a patient needs help, don't help him or her to disrobe. During an exam or treatment, if a brassiere must be unfastened or additional clothing must be removed, let the patient do it. If a patient *does* need help, then try to have it come from someone of the same gender—whether that is you or a staff person.

Uncovering the Patient. Expose only the portion of the patient's body on which you will be working—and don't uncover the patient without warning. Before the gown or drape is removed, the patient should know what will be removed, and why. Cover each area again before moving on to the next. If a gown or drape accidentally slips off the patient's shoulder or hip, replace it.

Using Common Sense. Don't have a patient strip bare so you can look at his or her left forearm. Instead have patients take off only the minimum of clothing. And, whenever possible, allow patients to leave on their underwear.

Communicating During Procedures

Don't Get Cute. To the patient, the use of slangy or humorous names for body parts may be suggestive or offensive. Besides, if something hurts, it isn't cute. A patient having foot problems, for instance, isn't likely to appreciate a reference to "tootsies."

Handle Humor With Care. Humor can be helpful in breaking the ice and improving communication—but don't use jokes that are sexual or suggestive, based on gender or ethnicity, or insulting to the patient. Steer clear of teasing, and keep the jokes strictly G-rated. Having trouble thinking of appropriate humor? Try the children's department of your local library.

Avoid Personal Comments. Compliments—even those that are innocently intended—may have the effect of sexualizing the doctor/patient relationship, because such comments are an integral part of the traditional courtship ritual. Personal comments while your hands are on the patient are particularly inappropriate; this is a time when communication should be at a minimum.

Control Your Gaze. Don't let your eyes wander to or linger on erogenous zones. It's not respectful, and if your patients catch you, your relationship with them could deteriorate rapidly. Ask yourself: Where does my gaze land, when I am looking at an attractive patient? Do my patients seem to notice? Even if no one seems to notice (and even if they do notice, most people will be too embarrassed to mention it), could this ever affect my ability to care for a patient?

Be Alert for Hidden Reservations. Always be sensitive to how patients respond to your requests for performing procedures. Listen not only to words, but also to tone of voice, and observe body language.

Get Feedback. Don't assume that your touch or other communication will have the effect that you intend; and don't assume that your hidden or even unconscious intentions will not be communicated to the patient.

DOCTOR-CENTERED INTERVENTIONS

Doctor-centered interventions include behavioral and educational interventions. They involve a personal/professional assessment on the part of the practitioner—an honest appraisal of attitudes and behavior—followed by any changes in attitudes and behavior that are indicated. Such interventions take time and willingness, and ideally will be part of an ongoing process of self-assessment and training of all doctors. The effects of personal and professional development are the most lasting. The benefit of doing such work may become evident immediately or after some time.

There are many ways to implement behavioral interventions; it can be done by making personal/professional changes, through training, through therapy, through professional supervision, and by working with a peer group or a buddy. For maximum safety, employ more than one of the above recommendations. Each has a different focus, and will shed light on behavior in different ways.

Behavioral Interventions

Avoid Sexual Behavior. Do not sexualize the relationship with your patient. "Sexualizing" is making a procedure or a conversation that is not implicitly sexual into something that is sexual or could be interpreted as being sexual. For example, using sexually charged slang words to refer to body parts can turn a discussion of a medical condition into something entirely different; and hugging, which can be an innocent human-to-human contact of greeting or comfort, also can become or can be taken for the prelude to a sexual act.

Respect Professional Boundaries. The relationship between doctor and patient is a fiduciary one; the practitioner has accepted the obligation to set aside his or her personal agenda and act only for the benefit of the patient. Such a relationship strictly limits the kinds of behavior that are acceptable within it. The doctor must honor these boundaries, even if they are ignored by the patient.

Do Not Ignore Sexual Feelings. Suppressing or denying sexual feelings toward a patient will not make such feelings go away; it will only make you less aware of how those feelings are affecting your relationship with that patient.

If repressed, an emotion or attraction is likely to go bubbling along out of sight, in your subconscious, like a tune that you don't even know you are humming. Without realizing it, you may spend extra time with certain patients whom you find attractive—or, if you fear involvement, you may slight them. You may say or do things you shouldn't. These problems are more readily managed or averted if you remain aware of your own feelings.

Do Not Indulge Sexual Feelings. A health-care practice is not a dating service. If you have little social life outside of the practice, heed the advice of the experts: Get a life.[2]

Never Ask Patients Out. A romantic or sexual relationship between doctor and patient is not appropriate, and generally is not legal.

Dismissing a patient so that the two of you can date also should be avoided. This is better than continuing to treat a patient and getting involved anyway—but it is not a cure-all.

Simply ending the doctor/patient relationship *does not* eliminate the possibility that sexual contact between a doctor and a former patient may be unethical. If, for instance, you use the patient's last visit to ask for a date or discuss your mutual interest in dating, it can later be said that the person was still a patient at the time of your discussion. Even after the patient has been dismissed, the former doctor/patient dynamic is apt to infuse any resulting personal relationship. The degree to which a particular patient is susceptible to such influence is something you are likely to learn only when it is too late.

If you still intend to do this, be aware: a waiting period of at least two years, is recommended—and for some professions, it is required. What is more, during this waiting period, there must be no office visits or reminders, no letters, no phone calls, and no other communication. The point, after all, is to *not* be continuing the existing relationship.

Avoid Dual Relationships. If one of your patients is also your dentist, or your carpenter, or your friend, then you have a dual relationship with this patient; and you may find that this creates difficulties that you are not prepared to handle. Keeping boundaries clear in such a relationship is not easy. Having a trained supervisor to consult about such a case could be very valuable.

Treat Patients Equally. A policy of uniform treatment of all patients protects everyone; it is an ideal to strive for. Making this a habit can prevent you from unconsciously slighting patients because they aren't attractive, or from giving them special treatment because they are attractive.[3]

Avoid or Minimize Hugging. Some doctors have gotten into the habit of saying hello by hugging their patients, but this is taking a liberty with another person's body. Forcing such an intimacy not only may drive some patients away and stop them from referring their friends or relatives, but may even lead them to warn people away from your practice. Many patients simply do not feel comfortable with hugging—even some of those who say yes, when asked if it is okay. Other patients could interpret the hugs that you intended as a friendly gesture as an indication that you are attracted to them. Be careful.

If you have been hugging your patients, evaluate this practice: Are you doing it for yourself, the patient, or both? Do you hug patients on every visit, or just occasionally? If you hug occasionally, then what is the occasion? Which patients do you hug—patients of the same sex? Of the opposite sex? Are patients asking to be hugged? Who initiates the hugs? Who ends them? What happens if you want a hug and the patient doesn't?

When a patient is distraught and needs or seeks comfort, or when a patient is feeling ecstatic about something that has just happened to them, a hug may be in order. But always ask first, and limit hugging to those patients you are certain want to be hugged. Never envelop the patient. Instead, open your arms and let the patient make the final approach. And keep any hugs crisp and short; this is, after all, a professional relationship.

Educational Interventions

Educational interventions include workshops and training programs, personal counseling or psychotherapy, professional supervision, peer-group supervision, "buddy system" supervision, and solitary explorations.

The Safe Practice Analysis, which is presented in the next chapter, offers another kind of educational intervention. It includes a set of questionnaires involving the doctor, the staff and the patients—as well as the buddy or supervisor, if such a relationship exists—in assessing the safety and comfort level of a health-care practice.

Workshops and Training Programs. Most training programs are either workshops or lectures.

In a workshop setting, everyone has an opportunity to hear the questions, comments, and concerns of others. Such a setting also allows for the sharing of information and experiences, in which participants can discover some of the most common pitfalls of practice. Many insights can be gained, which could become useful in the future. The workshop format also permits the use of role-playing exercises, in which participants can gain practice in dealing with a wide range of situations. The participants' own strengths and weaknesses become evident in the process.

Listening to a lecture does not allow for such involvement, although a lecture can be an efficient way of covering a large amount of material in a short period of time. The ideal format is a combination of a short lecture with lots of opportunities for active participation.

Subjects to explore include ethics, touch, gender, sexuality, sexual/professional boundaries, communication (honing listening and speaking skills, becoming more aware of non-verbal communication, and learning about the needs of patients and their communication styles), the changing doctor/patient relationship and the necessary skills for the new era we are now entering.

Examples of possible role-play topics include:

- A patient asks you out.
- You feel attracted to a patient.
- A patient is flirting with you.
- You wish to ask a patient out.
- You are in, or are considering, a dual relationship with a patient.

Benefits: Workshop settings yield many benefits. A lot of insights can be gained just through listening to the concerns, questions, and experiences of others. Activities can include role-playing, group discussion, listening to others and their concerns, and questions and solutions.

Drawbacks: Confidentiality is a realistic concern. There also are costs involved, sometimes including travel expenses.

Personal Therapy. Some doctors may desire to have an in-depth experience of personal exploration. With ongoing personal therapy, it is possible to delve into issues without fear of judgment and with total confidentiality.

Benefits: You may gain the ability to see patterns in your behavior; you will have the opportunity to explore attitudes and behavior with someone who is there to support your self-discovery.

Drawbacks: The cost is likely to be substantial, and a commitment to the process is required. It may take some time to find a therapist with whom you can establish a rapport. The discoveries that you make could cause a shake-up of your life and your practice.

Professional Supervision. In the mental-health fields, it is common practice for each doctor to have a supervisor. This supervisor is often a well-experienced and well-trained colleague with a therapy or consulting background. Physical health-care professionals would benefit from supervision, as well. The challenge will be to find such a qualified supervisor. At this time, the most likely candidates are psychotherapists, since few people in the physical health professions are trained or available to provide such mentoring.

Supervision can be one-on-one or in groups of practitioners. Meetings should be scheduled at regular intervals, so that problems can be nipped in the bud and so that, when questions arise, practitioners can promptly bring them up with their supervisor. This is an opportunity to look at all aspects of a problem, and to explore the ways in which the practitioner may be contributing to it. Supervision may involve speaking with the supervisor about difficulties, role-playing, listening together to taped conversations with patients, and discussing goals for working with particular patients, as well as addressing the practitioner's personal challenges as they come up in practice and with certain patients.

Attractions are one of the many kinds of difficulties that arise in practice, and having a knowledgeable supervisor to work with can be far superior to attempting to handle something so difficult alone. The rationalizations that might be used to deny that an attraction exists, or that it is a problem, are likely to collapse under the scrutiny of supervision, enabling you to recognize and address the problem.

Benefits: The one-on-one or small-group format allows for intensive personal exploration and challenge. When the relationship between supervisor and colleague is a good one, it is possible to grow much more quickly as a practitioner than when the practitioner tries to do it all alone.

Drawbacks: There may be substantial fees, especially for one-on-one supervision. In group supervision, there is less opportunity for confidentiality; in individual work, less opportunity for feedback from members of a group.

Peer-Group Supervision. In peer-group supervision, a group of motivated colleagues gets together approximately once a month to have discussions, do role-playing, interpret one another's difficulties in practice, and give advice or support as needed.

Benefits: In a group of peers, it may be possible to hear and see problems in others that one otherwise might have difficulty recognizing in oneself. There are more points of view, and a wider perspective, than with the buddy system. And there is little or no cost.

Drawbacks: There is less confidentiality than with either the buddy system or professional supervision. A group discussion easily can be dominated by one or two individuals. The system offers little time for any individual practitioner.

Buddy System. This system is as simple as it sounds: Two doctors pick one another as buddies. They make a contract to help one another for a specified period of time, a contract that can be renewed if both agree. They meet at regular intervals. And during stressful times, each buddy has the obligation to let the other know that something in his or her life or practice is out of balance and creating stress. The buddies will look out for each other.

Benefits: There is no cost, and easy availability. Ongoing mutual assistance is possible.

Drawbacks: There is a tendency to pick someone with whom you are comfortable with, someone a lot like you—someone who will think that everything you do is okay, even if it isn't. There might be a tendency to go easy on one another, with the result that criticisms are sugar-coated or not given at all.

Solitary Explorations. Ultimately, everything does comes down to needing to do it alone. Any change in attitude and behavior involves first seeing the need for change, and then being willing to make the necessary changes happen.

Benefits: This is the level at which all personal and professional development must occur. No one can change you but you.

Drawbacks: Everyone has blind spots. Without honest feedback from others, it may be difficult or impossible to identify the places where problems exist and change is needed. Solitary explorations therefore should be paired with at least one of the other explorations described above.

SUPERVISION—OR THE BUDDY SYSTEM—FOR SAFE PRACTICE

The Value of a Second Opinion

Doctors tend to become isolated, especially those in solo practice. Unless a practitioner makes a serious attempt to socialize, he or she may meet few people outside the practice. It is little wonder, therefore, that many physicians become entangled with patients, or that buddies and supervisors can be so valuable.

Outside the mental health-care fields, supervision is a new concept. Until recently, it was assumed that once they were licensed, health-care practitioners would forever be capable, honorable, and able to deal with anything that might arise in practice. It is unwise to believe that this is always true.

As the importance of supervision becomes more widely understood, we believe that it will come to be seen as an essential and integral part of practice.

Supervision vs. the Buddy System: How They Differ

Training. Supervisors are trained to deal with any personal issues that may arise; they are trained to work with people who are resisting and denying and in other ways avoiding looking at themselves. It's their job to promote growth. A supervisor is likely to be harder on you than a buddy.

Payment. A supervisory relationship involves payment to the supervisor. The buddy relationship involves an equal exchange of services with a colleague.

Background. A professional supervisor might be a psychotherapist, psychologist or social worker—or a health-care professional in your own profession or a similar profession who has experience working with colleagues. A buddy is likely to be a colleague from your own profession.

Personal and Practice Development. The supervisory relationship can allow for a level of development that is very difficult to attain on one's own, because people tend to see what they want to see and hear what they want to hear. A good buddy relationship can do the same. But in most cases, a buddy will be someone with whom you have a great deal in common; besides a profession, buddies are likely to share biases, blind spots, and rationalizations.

The Supervisory Relationship

PURPOSE: To obtain feedback from a trained observer—someone with no ties to your practice environment—about yourself and your practice. To determine to what degree you are creating a safe and comfortable environment for your patients and staff. To provide you with support and assistance as you make whatever changes are necessary. To help you deal with difficult decisions or crises that may arise in your practice.

How It Works. Supervision involves hiring a trained professional to provide help either in a one-on-one situation or for a small group.

The supervisory relationship involves personal analysis as well as practice support; it may challenge not only the way you practice but also many of your ideas and assumptions. To use this relationship to its fullest, you must approach it with total honesty and a willingness to really look at yourself. Within a healthy supervisory relationship, you will be able to be yourself. Ideally, you will feel safe enough to take an in-depth look at your strengths and weaknesses, agendas and motivations, challenges and victories.

The commitment to work together should be for a specified period of time; one year or longer is ideal.

What to Expect. The following guidelines apply equally to the buddy system and the supervisory relationship.

Honesty: Say what you feel, see, perceive, believe. The relationship is a vehicle for discussing your particular challenges in practice and in your personal life, particularly as they pertain to practice.

Communication: Speak at least once a month by phone. Meet once every month or every other month.

Getting to know you: The supervisor needs to know the supervisee well, including the his or her weak points, what is going on in his or her life—crises, changes, personal and professional relationships—and the stresses he or she is under.

Getting to know your practice: This includes the procedures used in your practice, the amount of touching, the amount of touching of bare skin, the office layout, the staff, the philosophy of patient care, gender attitudes, sexuality issues.

Experiencing your practice: The supervisor should be taken through the procedures that are used in the practice, so that he or she can point out any problems and indicate how procedures could be altered to provide more safety and comfort.

Growth: The supervisor's job is to promote the growth of the practitioner. The supervisee's job is to want to grow.

The Buddy Relationship

Friendship may be the best antidote for the alienation that is the inevitable result of corporate and professional styles of life.

—Sam Keen,
"Fire in the Belly," 1991

PURPOSE: To support, challenge and learn from one another, in order to provide the safest and most comfortable practice environment for both. To assist one another as the necessary changes are made. To help your buddy recognize and deal with problems as they arise.

How It Works. When two practitioners have agreed to team up and become "buddies," chances are that they like and respect each other. There is a plus and a minus to that. It can make it easier to allow yourself to be evaluated, but it also could make it more difficult. Doing the evaluating might be tough—after all, you are colleagues. This is the challenge, but it is worth the work of learning to become truly honest with each other.

The commitment to being buddies should not be taken lightly. The commitment should be for one year, and then should be renewed if it's working for both of you. If it's not working for one or both, then it's important to discuss that openly. There are pros and cons to working with the same buddy for a long period of time, as there are to having a series of different buddies.

The plus side of maintaining the same buddy over a period of time is, as you continue the buddy relationship, you may develop enough trust so that both of you can be honest without becoming enemies. The minus is that you may both become lazy, not looking too deeply at one another or challenging one another.

The plus to having different buddies is that you can get different kinds of feedback from each person. Also, by switching buddies from time to time, you will gain perspective. Some will notice things that others may not. Some may be more willing than others to express what they see and speak to you about it. The minus is that they will not know you so well.

What to Expect. The following are guidelines which apply equally to both the buddy system and the supervisor/supervisee relationship.

Honesty: If you are not both willing to be honest, you are wasting one another's time. Make the most of this opportunity to discuss your particular challenges in practice. Say what you feel, see, perceive.

Get to know one another: Each buddy should keep up with what is going on in the other's life—crises, changes, personal and professional relationships—as well as with the buddy's weak points and any stresses he or she may be under.

Communication: Speak at least once a month by phone. Meet once every one to two months.

Get to know the buddy's practice: This includes the procedures used in each practice, the amount of touching, the amount of touching of bare skin, the office layout, the staff, the philosophy of patient care, gender attitudes, sexuality issues.

Experience the buddy's practice: Each buddy should be taken through the procedures used in the other's practice, so that he or she can point out any problems and indicate how procedures could be altered to provide more safety and comfort. This also may be a chance for the visiting buddy to pick up tips about what works.

Growth: Ideally, such a relationship will promote growth for both parties.

NOTES

1.   For a lengthier discussion of draping procedures, see the section on physician and patient clothing in "Back to basics . . . The 'Slippery Slope': Boundary Issues for the Chiropractic Physician" by Linda J. Bowers, in *Topics in Clinical Chiropractic*: 1(3) 1994. Dr. Bowers is the chairwoman of the Diagnosis Department at the Northwestern College of Chiropractic, in Bloomington, Minn.

2. As John C. Gonsiorek puts it, "Maintaining a personal support system, an identity separate from one's profession, and a meaningful and varied life can be some of the best insurance . . . against boundary problems. Simply stated, get a life and keep a life." From his chapter entitled "Boundary Challenges When Both Therapist and Client Are Gay Males," in *Breach of Trust: Sexual Exploitation by Health Care Professionals and Clergy*, John C. Gonsiorek, ed. Thousand Oaks, Calif.: Sage Publications, Inc., 1995, 232.

3. K. Kitchner, "Dual Role Relationships: What Makes Them So Problematic? " *Journal of Counseling and Development*, 67 (1988), 217-221.

— *13* —

Safe Practice Analysis

PURPOSE: To determine whether and to what degree we and our staff may be insensitive, improper, or harmful in the care of patients.

WHAT IS THE SAFE PRACTICE ANALYSIS?

It is human nature to see what we want to see and to hear what we want to hear, and all of us have blind spots. Those are the reasons for the Safe Practice Analysis. It goes beyond the practitioner, asking staff, patients, and perhaps colleagues to also join in evaluating the practice. It asks important questions about patient care, about the doctor and staff, and about the general office environment. This analysis includes:

A Risk Factor Analysis

The Sexual Misconduct Risk Factor Analysis (RFA) poses specific questions about doctor attitudes and behaviors.

It can be self-scored, it requires little interpretation, and it can be kept private. The results give a practitioner a quick self-assessment of his or her current risk level for sexual misconduct, and can help to identify some of the riskiest behaviors.

The RFA can be used independently of the rest of the Safe Practice Assessment—but it is only a tool. Like any tool, it is—at best—only as good as the knowledge and skills of its user. The RFA requires both insight and honesty, it cannot see around the blind spots that each of us has, and it cannot detect the many risky behaviors that it does not specifically mention.

The RFA can be used as a periodic evaluation, to pinpoint times when your risk is particularly high, or it can be used together with the Practice Evaluation Questionnaires as part of the Safe Practice Analysis.

If you get a low score on the RFA, but have not done the remainder of the Safe Practice Analysis, please do not assume that you are safe. A low score indicates that you are not experiencing significant personal or professional stress, and that you *perceive* your behavior to be safe. However, even doctors who are guilty of some kinds of sexual misconduct may score low on this questionnaire if they believe their actions to be in the best interest of their patients.

Practice Evaluation Questionnaires

The Practice Evaluation Questionnaires, described below, contain general questions that are intended to determine how you can improve your practice, and how you can avoid making any grave mistakes in the area of sexual misconduct.

A Doctor Self-Evaluation Questionnaire. This questionnaire, to be filled out by the practitioner, is used to evaluate both the doctor and the staff. (Unlike the RFA, it is meant to be shown to others for feedback.)

A Staff Evaluation Questionnaire. This questionnaire, to be filled out by staff members, is used to evaluate both the doctor and the staff.

A Buddy/Supervisor Questionnaire: This questionnaire enlists the assistance of someone from outside the office environment—someone who can provide a second opinion on the way the practice operates. A "buddy" is a colleague you have agreed to work with, for the express purpose of guiding and supporting each other. A "supervisor" is either a psychotherapist or a colleague—from your profession or a related profession—who is trained to work with colleagues.

A Patient Evaluation Questionnaire. This questionnaire, presented in two versions, asks active and inactive patients to help evaluate the practice.

Instructions for Analyzing the Results

Each questionnaire is accompanied by directions and suggestions for how to handle both the evaluation and the analysis. The goal is to enable you to find out whether the office environment you are creating is safe for everyone—the doctor, the patients, and the staff—and to discover to what degree your patients are satisfied.

Putting It All Together

This section, which begins on page 151, includes instructions on how to tabulate the results of the Practice Evaluation Questionnaires; advice on how to distinguish among Highest Risk, High Risk, and Lower Risk problems; and an explanation of how to compare the results of the RFA and the Practice Evaluation Questionnaires.

WHY DO THE PRACTICE ANALYSIS?

To Ensure a Safe Practice

By using all of the questionnaires, you will discover, from varying sources, whether you are being as sensitive and as appropriate as you need to be with all your patients. If one or more of your behaviors are offensive or even harmful, it is better to learn about that *before* complaints are filed against you. Formal complaints are not the best way to find out that you are doing something that patients don't like; proactivity is much more sensible.

To Ensure Satisfied Patients

The patient questionnaires enable you to determine the level of patient satisfaction with your practice. And, you will discover exactly what it is that your patients are satisfied and not satisfied with. Satisfied patients, as we know, are more likely to get better, more likely to stay with a practice, more likely to refer other patients, and in general, are likely to make practice a much more enjoyable experience.

In their book, *A Complaint Is a Gift*, Janelle Barlow and Claus Moller write that customer complaints can be a valuable strategic marketing tool. A complaint, they note, is a statement that a customer's expectations haven't been met. And even in the business world, they say, only one in twenty-seven dissatisfied customers actually complains.

So, if you receive one patient complaint of any kind, there are probably dozens of other patients who are dissatisfied. Some of the complaints you'll be receiving from patients aren't the sort that would bring you into the court-room—but avoiding litigation shouldn't be your only goal; creating patient satisfaction is important, too.

SEXUAL MISCONDUCT RISK FACTOR ANALYSIS

> PURPOSE: The Risk Factor Analysis (RFA) is a tool that can be used to quickly evaluate your current risk level for sexual misconduct.

This questionnaire was created by Ben Benjamin, Ph.D., and Angelica Redleaf, D.C.; some portions are adapted from the article "Are You In Trouble With A Client?" by Estelle Disch, Ph.D., which appeared in *Massage Therapy Journal*, Summer 1992. Ben Benjamin is the director of the Muscular Therapy Institute in Cambridge, Mass. Estelle Disch has practiced for more than 20 years as a clinical sociologist and psychotherapist in Boston, Mass., and is the co-director of BASTA! (Boston Associates to Stop Therapy Abuse).

What is the Risk Factor Analysis?

The RFA asks very specific questions. Some are about stress you may be experiencing in your life or in your practice. Others are about attractions to patients, interactions with patients, and attitudes toward patients. The questions are based on typical kinds of doctor behaviors and attitudes.

The RFA is meant for you to keep to yourself. It can be taken again from time to time—for example, every six months—to give you a quick idea of your risk level. It can be used independently of the Practice Analysis, which includes more general questions about doctor and staff behavior and attitudes.

How Does the RFA Differ from the Doctor Self-Analysis?

The RFA and the Doctor Self-Evaluation Questionnaire (DSE) both ask the practitioner to self-evaluate his or her level of risk. The DSE asks general questions about your behaviors, attitudes, skills, and attributes, and about your staff's behaviors, skills, and attitudes. The RFA asks very specific questions that are designed to give you a quick idea of the level of risk you are incurring by practicing the way that you do.

By comparing your responses to both questionnaires (see page 158), you will be able to gain a very clear picture of what *you think* about yourself as a practitioner, and of what *you think* about your staff. This information is a good start, but neither of these self-evaluations can see past your own blind spots.

The rest of the Practice Analysis will either confirm, challenge, or illuminate your ideas about yourself as a practitioner, and about your practice as a whole.

Instructions

Place a check-mark next to the number (1, 2, or 3) of each statement that applies to you. When you have completed the questionnaire, add up all of the numbers that are the same—i.e., add up all the number 1s on a page and write that number at the bottom of each sheet, then do the same for all the 2s and 3s on each sheet. Add up the totals for each number on the last page in the space provided. Directions for assessing *your* RFA numbers are on the next page.

At the end of the self-scoring section, there are guidelines for comparing your RFA results with the results of the Doctor Self-Evaluation and the rest of the Practice Analysis.

RISK FACTOR ANALYSIS QUESTIONNAIRE

1   I want this patient to like me.

1   I like it when my patients find me attractive. I keep this to myself.

2   Sometimes I schedule the patients that I really like last so that I can spend more time with them.

2   I am surprised by how much I anticipate this patient's visit.

2   I think about this patient frequently.

1   I have not been in a relationship in a long time.

1   I feel lonely much of the time, unless I'm working.

2   With certain patients I have trouble asking to be paid.

1   I talk about my personal life to my patients.

2   I find myself working weekends to accommodate a few patients I like.

1   Some of my patients rely on me a lot.

2   I feel as if I am under tremendous pressure.

1   I like it when my patients look up to me.

2   I feel like I have very little to give lately.

2   My relationship with my significant other(s) isn't meeting my needs.

3   I've sometimes touched patients in inappropriate ways.

3   I've had sex with patients.

3   I've had sex with patients in the office.

2   I dress particularly well when I know one or more of my patients has an appointment that day.

1   I fantasize about what it would be like to have sex with some of my patients.

2   I'm not charging one or more of the patients to whom I'm attracted.

2   I have some of my patients take off more of their clothes than they really need to remove.

2   I sometimes sneak looks as patients are undressing.

2   I believe it's okay to date my patients.

2   I sometimes tell dirty jokes to my patients.

2   I like doing treatments in those areas of patient's bodies that are close to their erogenous zones.

2   I compliment patients when I think they look nice.

1   This patient feels more like a friend.

2   I often tell my personal problems to one or more of my patients.

2   I feel sexually aroused by one or more of my patients.

3   I'm waiting to dismiss this patient so that we can become romantically involved.

2   To be honest, I think that good-bye hugs last too long with one or more of my patients.

2   Appointments with one or more of my patients last longer than with others.

2   I tend to accept gifts or favors from this patient without examining why a gift was given.

Totals for this page:

1 _____   2 _____   3 _____

1	I feel totally comfortable socializing with patients.
1	I have a barter arrangement with one or more of my patients that is sometimes a source of tension.
3	I have had sexual contact with one or more of my patients.
2	I have attended professional or social events at which I knew that this patient would be present.
2	This patient often invites me to social events and I don't feel comfortable saying either yes or no.
2	Sometimes when I'm working on this patient, I feel like the contact is sexualized for myself and maybe for the patient.
2	There's something I like about being alone in the office with this patient when no one else is around.
2	I am tempted to lock the door when working with this patient.
3	This patient is very seductive and I don't always know how to handle it.
2	I have invited this patient to public or social events.
1	I find myself cajoling, teasing, joking a lot with this patient.
3	I allow this patient to comfort me.
3	Sometimes I feel like I'm in over my head with this patient.
2	I feel overly protective of this patient.
3	I sometimes have a drink or use some recreational drug with this patient.
3	I am doing more for this patient than I would for any other patient.
2	I find it difficult to keep from talking about this patient with other people who are close to me.
2	I find myself saying a lot about myself with this patient—telling stories, engaging in peer-like conversation.
3	If I were to list patients with whom I could envision myself in a sexual relationship, this patient would be on the list.
3	I call this patient a lot and go out of my way to meet with him/her in locations convenient to him/her.
2	This patient has spent time at my home.
3	I often tell my personal problems to this patient.
3	I enjoy exercising my power over some of my patients.
3	I'm going through a crisis at this point in my life.
2	Sometimes I'm afraid I might burn out.
3	I need someone to take care of *me*.
3	If a patient consents to sex, it's okay.

Totals for this page:

1 _____   2 _____   3 _____

Totals for both pages:

1 _____   2 _____   3 _____

If you have checked off even one number 3: You are at risk. Know that you are a ticking time bomb who could potentially hurt yourself, your patient(s) and your profession! You would be very wise to get help from a therapist, consultant or significant other. You also should consider getting training in this area. Ignoring your high risk or attempting to get through this by yourself might be very unwise.

If you have checked off more than three number 2s: You have the potential for problems. The more number 2s you check off, the more your risk factor increases. You could use some help in getting yourself on track concerning professional boundaries.

If you checked off more than five number 1s: You may be overstepping your professional boundaries. You might not be in danger of overstepping them sexually, but you still could find yourself losing your effectiveness as a health provider. Be aware of your attitudes about patients, yourself, and your practice.

During times of stress and personal loss, we are more likely to overstep our professional boundaries. There are training sessions available that address the questions of boundaries and sexual misconduct, and there are therapists, mentors, friends, and colleagues who could help you at such times. Your risk is greatest when you attempt to go through such a transition all by yourself.

THE PRACTICE EVALUATION QUESTIONNAIRES

Doctor Self-Evaluation

PURPOSE: The DSE is one of the crucial steps of the overall Safe Practice Analysis, which is designed to determine to what degree you are creating a safe and comfortable practice environment, for yourself, your staff, and your patients.

Unlike the RFA, the DSE questions you in depth about your personal behavior with patients, your attitudes about them and your attitudes about yourself. There also are questions about how you perceive your staff's attitudes and behaviors.

This evaluation is meant to be shown to others whom you trust to be objective about the way you see yourself as practicing. It can be taken once a year, as part of the Practice Analysis, or it can be taken separately, whenever you are questioning your care of patients.

Remember, there are no wrong answers. The point of this questionnaire is to learn more about the way you practice and to identify areas of weakness. Any honest answer is the right answer.

DOCTOR SELF-EVALUATION QUESTIONNAIRE

PART I: These questions are about the way you see yourself and the way you practice.

1. Are you aware of anything that you do that seems to make your patients or staff feel unwelcome, uncomfortable, or unsafe? If so, how could that be changed?
EXPLAIN:

2. Do you believe that you have ever been sexually inappropriate with patients? staff?
EXPLAIN:

3. Do you ever feel you are taking risks with patients? Minimal? Moderate? Great?
EXPLAIN:

4. Do you ever touch patients in ways that might be considered inappropriate?
EXPLAIN:

5. Is there any office procedure that you believe could be altered or eliminated to provide a safer and more comfortable environment for patient, doctor, or staff?
EXPLAIN:

6. Would you feel capable of caring for a patient who you know has been previously sexually abused, either by another doctor or by some other person?
EXPLAIN:

7. Do you ever tell off-color jokes in the office? Do you ever use sexually charged terms when speaking with patients?
EXPLAIN:

8. What is your gender? Do you see it as a problem, or a potential problem?
EXPLAIN:

9. What is your sexual orientation? Do you see it as a problem, or a potential problem?
EXPLAIN:

10. Do you consider yourself to be very sexual? Somewhat sexual? Mildly sexual?
EXPLAIN:

11. Do you treat patients equally, regardless of their gender or their sexual orientation?
EXPLAIN:

12. Are you ever made uncomfortable by a patient's sexuality or sexual orientation? Has this ever made it difficult to care for a particular patient? How? What did you do?
EXPLAIN:

13. What is your marital status? Do you ever see it as a problem, or a potential problem?
EXPLAIN:

14. Are you especially attractive? Do you see this as a problem or potential problem?
EXPLAIN:

15. Do you treat patients differently if they are attractive? Single? Both?
EXPLAIN:

16. Are there any patients to whom you give special attention, or for whom you bend office rules?
EXPLAIN:

17. Have patients ever expressed an interest in you on a personal/dating level? If yes, how did you feel about it? If no, how did you feel about it?
EXPLAIN:

18. Are you affectionate? Outgoing? Flirtatious? Is this ever a problem, or a potential problem? Could this generate special interest, or seem to indicate special interest?
EXPLAIN:

19. Do you feel you can get away with bending rules, because you can handle it?
EXPLAIN:

20. Do you make immediate notes of every office visit, including a description of any unusual, unsettling or inappropriate behavior on your part or a patient's part?
EXPLAIN:

Part II: These questions are for you to answer about your staff.

1. Are you aware of anything that staff members do that seems to make patients or staff feel unwelcome, uncomfortable, or unsafe? If so, how could that be changed?
EXPLAIN:

2. Do staff members ever act in sexually inappropriate ways with patients?
EXPLAIN:

3. Do staff members touch patients as part of their work? Because they choose to?
EXPLAIN:

4. Do staff members touch patients only in ways that are respectful and appropriate?
EXPLAIN:

5. Is there anything any staff member generally does that could be altered or eliminated to provide a safer and more comfortable environment for patients, doctor, or staff?
EXPLAIN:

6. Do you feel that the staff would be capable of interacting with and caring for a patient who has been previously sexually abused, by another doctor or by some other person?
EXPLAIN:

7. Do staff members ever tell off-color jokes in the office?
EXPLAIN:

8. Do staff members ever use sexually charged terms when speaking with patients? with the doctor(s)? with other staff members?
EXPLAIN:

9. Are any staff members uncomfortable about patients who are homosexual or bisexual?
EXPLAIN:

10. Does any staff member's sexuality ever create problems in the office?
EXPLAIN:

11. Do the staff members treat patients equally, whatever their gender or sexual orientation?
EXPLAIN:

12. Are staff members ever uncomfortable about a patient's sexuality or sexual orientation? Does this ever make it difficult for them to deal with a patient? How?
EXPLAIN:

13. Do any staff members have difficulty dealing with people who are very open about their sexuality? With people who are very shy or private about their sexuality?
EXPLAIN:

14. Are any staff members especially attractive? Is this a problem or potential problem?
EXPLAIN:

15. Do any staff members treat patients differently if they are attractive? Single? Both?
EXPLAIN:

16. Are there any patients to whom the staff members give special attention, or who the staff let break office rules?
EXPLAIN:

17. Have patients ever expressed an interest in any staff member on a personal/dating level? If yes, how did the staff feel about it? If no, how did the staff feel about it?
EXPLAIN:

18. Is any staff member very affectionate? Outgoing? Flirtatious? Is this a problem, or a potential problem? Could it generate special interest in this staff member, or seem to indicate special interest by this staff member?
EXPLAIN:

19. Does any staff member feel it's okay to bend rules, because he or she can handle it?
EXPLAIN:

20. What problems do patients present for the staff?
EXPLAIN:

Analyzing Your Questionnaire. Remember, there are no wrong answers. The point of this questionnaire is to learn about the way you practice and to identify weak areas. Any honest answer is the right answer.

The maximum benefits are derived from this questionnaire when you ask others to read your responses to it, compare your responses with the responses of your patients and staff on the questionnaires that follow, and ask for their opinions about how you see yourself and your practice. Ask those who are nearest to you on a day-to-day basis to help with this. Tell them to be completely honest. Expect comments and criticisms; that is what you are asking them to provide. Do not take their responses as anything other than help. If you find yourself defending yourself with ''But I . . . ,'' then pay close attention.

Possible Warning Signs. If there is any indication in your questionnaire of problems that involve sexuality, gender, touch, consent, or a lack of respect for patients, circle those answers in red. They represent potentially high-risk behaviors or attitudes that must not be ignored. Share your completed DSE questionnaire with a colleague, friend, therapist, or trusted staff member, for discussion and feedback. (This is a good idea, in any case.) Be on the lookout for related high-risk behaviors and attitudes as you continue practicing. Make a decision about how you can change these risky behaviors or attitudes.

What you and others should look for, in reviewing your questionnaire:

- Any signs of defensiveness.
- Any lack of willingness to answer completely and honestly.
- Any question to which the response was a false answer or no answer.
- Any answers indicating a possible lack of professionalism.
- Anything that makes anyone uncomfortable; that means it needs a closer look.
- Any indication of a lack of respect, for anyone or everyone.
- Any differences between your assessment of yourself or your practice and the way you and your practice are seen by others.

The Staff Evaluation

Your doctor(s) need(s) your help. The doctor(s) must know to what degree everyone in the office—especially the doctor—is creating a safe and comfortable environment for patients. Patients are more and more sensitive to behavior and attitudes on the part of doctor and staff that are inappropriate, offensive, or even harmful. If they don't like the way they are being treated, they often don't just go elsewhere, they speak out. As a result, doctors are increasingly being accused of sexual misconduct. The office environment must be a safe and comfortable place in which even the most sensitive patient will feel secure.

It has become clear to your doctor(s) that it is time to deal with this critical issue in practice. Please fill out the following questionnaire as honestly as you possibly can. You are a part of the health-care team in this office, and as a result, you have information and feelings that will be extremely valuable. There are questions about the attitudes and behaviors of the doctor(s), about your attitudes and behaviors, and about the other staff.

The doctor(s) will see your responses. They have been warned to be open and receptive to your comments and criticisms, because to improve the practice, they must know what you see and what you perceive. Please be honest.

STAFF EVALUATION QUESTIONNAIRE

PART I: These questions are about the way you see your doctor or doctors.

1. Is there anything the doctor does that makes patients or staff feel unwelcome or unsafe? If so, how could that be changed?
EXPLAIN:

2. Has the doctor ever acted in sexually inappropriate ways with patients? With other staff? With you?
EXPLAIN:

3. Do you ever think the doctor is taking risks with patients? How big are the risks? Minimal? Moderate? Great?
EXPLAIN:

4. Is the doctor always respectful and appropriate when he or she touches patients?
EXPLAIN:

5. Is there any office procedure that you believe could be altered or eliminated to provide a safer and more comfortable environment for patient, doctor, or staff?
EXPLAIN:

6. Would an individual who has been sexually abused, either by another doctor or some other person, be able to feel safe and comfortable as a patient of the doctor?
EXPLAIN:

7. Does the doctor ever tell off-color jokes in the office? Does he or she ever use sexually charged terms when speaking with patients?
EXPLAIN:

8. Whatever the doctor's gender (male or female), could it be or has it been a problem?
EXPLAIN:

9. Whatever the doctor's sexual orientation, could it be or has it been a problem?
EXPLAIN:

10. How sexual does the doctor seem? Very? Somewhat? Mildly? Is this a problem?
EXPLAIN:

11. Does the doctor treat patients equally, regardless of gender or sexual orientation?
EXPLAIN:

12. Does the doctor ever seem uncomfortable about a patient's sexuality or sexual orientation? Has this ever affected a patient's care? How? What did the doctor do?
EXPLAIN:

13. Do you know the doctor's marital status? Could it be, or has it been, a problem?
EXPLAIN:

14. Is the doctor attractive? Do you see this as a problem or potential problem?
EXPLAIN:

15. Does the doctor treat patients differently if they are attractive? Single? Both?
EXPLAIN:

16. Does the doctor give any patients special attention, or bend office rules for them?
EXPLAIN:

17. Have patients ever expressed an interest in the doctor on a personal or dating level?
Has the doctor ever dated a patient?
EXPLAIN:

18. Is the doctor affectionate? Outgoing? Flirtatious? Have patients ever thought, or
could they think, that this indicates special interest? Does it generate special interest?
EXPLAIN:

19. Does the doctor tend to make rules, but not follow them?
EXPLAIN:

20. Would you feel comfortable sending your daughter or son (if you have one) to the
doctor? Your mother or father? Why?
EXPLAIN:

PART II: These questions are about the way you see yourself and other staff.

1. Is there anything you or other staff members do that seems to make patients, doctors,
or staff feel unwelcome, uncomfortable or unsafe? If so, how could that be changed?
EXPLAIN:

2. Do you or other staff members ever act in sexually inappropriate ways with patients?
Doctors? Staff?
EXPLAIN:

3. Do you and other staff touch patients? As part of your work? Because you like to?
EXPLAIN:

4. Do you and other staff touch patients only in ways that are respectful and appropriate?
EXPLAIN:

5. Is there anything you and other staff do that you believe could be altered or eliminated
to provide a safer and more comfortable environment for patient, doctor or staff?
EXPLAIN:

6. Would you and other staff be capable of interacting with and caring for a patient who
has been previously sexually abused, by another doctor or by some other person?
EXPLAIN:

7. Do you or other staff members ever tell off-color jokes in the office?
EXPLAIN:

8. Do you or other staff members ever use sexually charged terms when speaking with
patients? With the doctor or doctors? With other staff members?
EXPLAIN:

9. Are you or other staff uncomfortable about patients who are homosexual or bisexual?
EXPLAIN:

10. Does your sexuality, or another staff member's, ever create problems in the office?
EXPLAIN:

11. Do you and other staff members treat patients equally, whatever their gender or sexual orientation?
EXPLAIN:

12. Are you or other staff ever made uncomfortable by a patient's sexuality or sexual orientation? Has this ever made it difficult to deal with a particular patient? How?
EXPLAIN:

13. Do you or other staff members have difficulty dealing with people who are very open about their sexuality? With people who are very shy or private about their sexuality?
EXPLAIN:

14. Are you especially attractive, or is some other staff member? Is this a problem or potential problem?
EXPLAIN:

15. Do you or other staff treat patients differently if they are attractive? Single? Both?
EXPLAIN:

16. Are there any patients to whom you or other staff members give special attention, or who you let break office rules?
EXPLAIN:

17. Have patients ever expressed an interest in you or in other staff members on a personal or dating level? How do you feel about that?
EXPLAIN:

18. Are you or other staff affectionate? Outgoing? Flirtatious? Is this a problem, or a potential problem? Could it cause special interest, or seem to indicate special interest?
EXPLAIN:

19. Do you or other staff feel it's okay to bend rules, because you can handle it?
EXPLAIN:

20. What difficulties do patients present for you and other staff members?
EXPLAIN:

Thank you for your honesty and for your time in filling this out!

Analyzing the Staff Questionnaires. Be prepared for a wide range of responses from your staff. One staff member might be concerned about losing his or her job; another might be the kind of person who doesn't want to hurt anyone's feelings; another might see this as an opportunity to get back at you—or a coworker—or as a chance to vent some anger, frustration, or other emotion. The usefulness of their comments may vary, for those reasons. But, if the people on your staff have been completely honest, and if you can deal with their comments, this could be the ultimate source of feedback. You know them, and they know you.

Be sure to consult the section Putting It All Together (page 151) for more detailed information on analyzing the results—and to learn more about what sorts of comments can be discounted and what may be cause for immediate concern.

Buddy/Supervisor Evaluation

Under the buddy system, two doctors choose one another as buddies, agreeing to help one another for a specified period of time. The two parties look out for one another. This is an excellent, low-cost opportunity for both to obtain feedback on and monitoring of their practices. To make the system work, however, the participants need to be forthright and honest in their evaluations, resisting the temptation to whitewash their findings in the name of friendship or professional courtesy. A little diplomacy may also be required.

The questionnaire on the following pages is designed to help doctors who are buddies to carry out an honest, fair, and effective evaluation of one another.

An alternative to the buddy system is professional supervision. This is a more formal arrangement in which the doctor hires a fellow professional who has undergone special training, or a trained psychotherapist, to evaluate and monitor his or her practice.

The Buddy/Supervisor Evaluation—in fact, the entire Safe Practice Analysis—also can be used by professional supervisors as a part of this ongoing relationship.

BUDDY / SUPERVISOR QUESTIONNAIRE

PART I: These questions are about the doctor and the way he or she practices.

1. Is there anything you have observed the doctor doing, or have heard that the doctor does, that makes the patients or staff feel unwelcome, uncomfortable, or unsafe? If so, how could that be changed?
EXPLAIN.

2. Are you aware of the doctor having been sexually inappropriate with patients? Staff?
EXPLAIN.

3. Do you think the doctor is taking risks with patients? Minimal? Moderate? Great?
EXPLAIN.

4. Does the doctor ever appear to be inappropriate or disrespectful in his or her use of touch with patients? What kinds of touch have you observed or personally experienced the doctor using: Clinical? Nurturing? Sexual? Other?
EXPLAIN.

5. Is there any office procedure that you believe could be altered or eliminated to provide a safer and more comfortable environment for patient, doctor or staff?
EXPLAIN.

6. Do you think the doctor would be comfortable with and able to care for a patient who had been sexually abused, either by another doctor or by some other person?
EXPLAIN.

7. Does the doctor tell off-color jokes in the office? Does he or she use sexually charged terms or inappropriate sexual references in speaking with patients?
EXPLAIN.

8. Whatever the doctor's gender, does it seem to be a problem? Could it ever become a problem?
EXPLAIN.

9. Whatever the doctor's sexual orientation, does that orientation seem to be a problem? Could it ever become a problem?
EXPLAIN.

10. Does the doctor seem to be very sexual? Somewhat? Mildly? Do you see this as a problem or potential problem for the doctor's practice?
EXPLAIN.

11. Does the doctor treat patients equally, regardless of gender or sexual orientation?
EXPLAIN.

12. Is the doctor ever uncomfortable about a patient's sexuality or sexual orientation? Do you see this as a problem or potential problem? Could it ever affect patient care?
EXPLAIN.

13. Do patients seem to be aware of the doctor's marital status? Does it ever appear to be a problem, or a potential problem?
EXPLAIN.

14. Is the doctor attractive? Does the doctor seem to consider himself or herself to be attractive? Do you see this as a problem or potential problem?
EXPLAIN.

15. Does the doctor treat patients differently if they are attractive? Single? Both?
EXPLAIN.

16. Do there seem to be any patients to whom the doctor gives special attention, or for whom the doctor will bend office rules?
EXPLAIN.

17. To your knowledge, do patients ever express an interest in the doctor on a personal or dating level? Has the doctor ever dated a patient?
EXPLAIN.

18. Is the doctor affectionate? Outgoing? Flirtatious? Have patients ever thought, or could they think, that this indicates special interest? Does it generate special interest?
EXPLAIN.

19. Does the doctor make rules but not follow them? Does the doctor seem to feel entitled to bend rules, because he or she is strong or can handle it?
EXPLAIN.

20. Does the doctor make immediate notes of every office visit, including a description of any unusual, unsettling, or inappropriate behavior by doctor or patient? Does he or she promptly record the findings (positive or negative) of every exam?
EXPLAIN.

PART II: These are questions regarding the doctor's staff.

1. Are you aware of anything that staff members do that seems to make patients or staff feel unwelcome, uncomfortable or unsafe? If so, how could that be changed?
EXPLAIN.

2. Do staff members ever act in sexually inappropriate ways with patients?
EXPLAIN.

3. Do staff members touch patients as part of their work? Because they choose to?
EXPLAIN.

4. Do staff members touch patients only in ways that are respectful and appropriate?
EXPLAIN.

5. Is there anything any staff member generally does that could be altered or eliminated to provide a safer and more comfortable environment for patients, doctor, or other staff?
EXPLAIN.

6. Do you feel that the staff would be capable of interacting with and caring for a patient who has been previously sexually abused, by another doctor or by some other person?
EXPLAIN.

7. Do staff members ever tell off-color jokes in the office?
EXPLAIN.

8. Do staff members ever use sexually charged terms when speaking with patients? With

the doctor or doctors? With other staff members?
EXPLAIN.

9. Are any staff members uncomfortable about patients who are homosexual or bisexual?
EXPLAIN.

10. Does any staff member's sexuality ever create problems in the office?
EXPLAIN.

11. Do the staff members treat patients equally, whatever the patients' gender or sexual orientation?
EXPLAIN.

12. Are staff members ever made uncomfortable by a patient's sexuality or sexual orientation? Does this ever make it difficult for them to deal with a particular patient?
EXPLAIN.

13. Do any staff members have difficulty dealing with people who are very open about their sexuality? With people who are very shy or private about their sexuality?
EXPLAIN.

14. Are any members of the staff especially attractive? Does this seem to be a problem or potential problem?
EXPLAIN.

15. Do any staff members treat patients differently if they are attractive? Single? Both?
EXPLAIN.

16. Are there any patients to whom the staff give special attention, or for whom the staff will break office rules?
EXPLAIN.

17. Have patients ever expressed an interest in any staff member on a personal or dating level? If no, how does the staff feel about it? If yes, how did that staff member feel about it? What about his or her coworkers?
EXPLAIN.

18. Are any staff members especially affectionate? Outgoing? Flirtatious? Is this ever a problem, or a potential problem? Could it generate special interest, or seem to indicate special interest?
EXPLAIN.

19. Does any member of the staff seem to feel that it's okay to bend rules, because he or she knows the ropes or can handle it?
EXPLAIN.

20. Do staff members greet patients promptly? Do they answer the patients' questions or find someone who can?
EXPLAIN.

Analyzing the Results. The buddy or supervisor should analyze this questionnaire—organizing the comments, looking for patterns, and identifying problems—and then should schedule a meeting with the other doctor to go over the results together. This approach is far more effective than just filling out the form and handing it to the doctor. For instance, yes, you should tell the doctor if he or she seems to be groping the patients when doing a physical examination—but that's not the way to say it.

Emotionally loaded words are fine for your notes, if that's faster for you—but don't let anyone else see that version. Before going over your report with the doctor or with anyone else, rewrite it on another form. The revised version should still describe everything that you observed, but it should be stated in such a way that your report could be handed in to a high school English teacher, or printed in the local newspaper. Even the riskiest behavior can be described in dry terms that will make your buddy or supervisee more likely to listen and less likely to explode.

Begin by organizing your responses into the following categories. Using a separate sheet of ruled paper for each category, copy each comment you have made on the questionnaire onto a single line on the appropriate sheet or sheets. This makes it easier to spot patterns. Also, if you pass along an edited copy of these sheets, it will make it easier for the doctor to compare your responses with the results of the other Practice Evaluation Questionnaires. The categories are:

- doctor attributes
- doctor attitudes
- doctor behaviors
- doctor skills
- staff attitudes
- staff behaviors
- staff skills
- office environment
- office procedures

Next, look for patterns. You may find that many of your comments are related. For example:

- There may be a pattern of problems with touch or communication.
- Looking more deeply, you may find that this pattern indicates problems with power and a lack of respectful care, or problems with the obtaining of patient consent.
- There may be a pattern of difficulties with patients of a particular gender, which might indicate a problem with doctor attitudes toward that gender or a need to learn to better understand that gender's communication style.
- There could be a pattern of problems with patients of a particular age group or socioeconomic class; this could indicate problems in the way the doctor handles power or a lack of flexibility in his or her communication style.
- Sexually inappropriate comments or behavior may indicate that the doctor lacks awareness about what is appropriate, or lacks awareness of his or her own sexuality.
- A pattern of risky or out-of-character behavior, or of getting too personal with the

patients, might hint at boundary problems. Or, it might be a sign of a personal or professional crisis that is adversely affecting the way the doctor practices.

Finally, make notes for yourself, organize the material, and decide how to present your comments and suggestions. Then schedule a meeting, after hours or on a day off, at which you can present your findings and discuss them with your buddy or supervisee.

If there are many problems, or if some of them are very serious, determine which problems you will need to communicate right away—for instance, any problem or problems that have the potential to create legal difficulties. Go back over your comments—paying especial attention to those involving issues of sexuality, gender, touch, or lack of respect—and if any of them seem to indicate High Risk or Highest Risk problems (see page 155), circle those in red.

Any urgent or serious problems should be addressed at the first meeting with your buddy or supervisee; at later meetings, the two of you can concentrate on one problem at a time, in more depth. Less-urgent and lower-risk problems may be left for later. But before putting them aside, consider whether they could be related to the more urgent or more serious problems. And recognize that even if they are not major, these problems may be driving patients away.

When you meet with your buddy or supervisee, be careful in how you let him or her know what you have seen, heard, and felt. If possible, use the sandwich approach: Give a compliment, then the criticism, then another compliment. And at each meeting, try to stay focused on one problem or one related set of problems.

Receiving the Results. When you have an appointment to go over what your buddy/supervisor has found, prepare yourself. You may hear things you don't really want to hear.

Your buddy may be reluctant to hurt, anger, or offend. He or she may just be trying to be nice, and offer little or no outright criticism. (Your supervisor will have experience delivering comments, and will do it in a way that will hopefully have you feeling positive and encouraged). Listen carefully to what your buddy or supervisor does say and how he or she says it. If you think that your buddy is being too easy on you, and not being honest, go ahead and challenge him or her. Say, for example, "I don't believe you're being completely honest. Are you trying to protect my feelings? We're doing this in order to make sure that we're not harming our patients. Tell me the truth."

When criticized, don't fly off the handle, even if you think that the buddy or supervisor went overboard. He or she is just trying to do the job that you asked him or her to do. Look for the kernel of truth—the problem. When you think you've picked it out, confirm it with your buddy.

Once you've been told there is something that needs to be changed in your attitude or behavior, there are a few possibilities:

a. You have heard similar comments from more than one source, and you are convinced that there is a problem: Correct the problem.

b. You haven't heard the same thing from anyone else, but you agree that there's a problem: Correct the problem.

c. You disagree with the criticism, and others do also: Evaluate the criticism carefully—it still may be accurate. Consider seeking more feedback.

d. You disagree with the criticism, but you have heard similar comments from more than one source: Be prepared to reconsider. This almost certainly indicates that there is a problem, but it is in one of your blind spots.

Even if you remain unconvinced that there is a problem, consider making some adjustments in the way you practice. The goal, after all, is not to win a debate but to reduce the likelihood of creating dissatisfaction or giving offense.

The Patient Evaluation

In conducting any survey of patient satisfaction, it is important to contact both current and inactive patients. Satisfied patients, after all, are the most likely to stay with a practice, and dissatisfied patients are the most likely to leave. This is an opportunity to find out how you and your practice are doing, and in the process, to determine whether you and your staff are using any behavior or office practices that are inappropriate.

The Questionnaire. The same questionnaire can be used for both active patients and inactive patients. It has been designed to elicit patients' comments on a number of issues, without encouraging them to think that something may be wrong with the care that they have received. In the case of inactive patients, it also may serve to remind them of you.

The Cover Letter. The questionnaire itself should be accompanied by a letter explaining why you are asking people to answer these questions. Your signature on each letter is a nice touch, when you are asking patients to give you their time and their opinions. Two sample letters are included, one for active patients and one for inactive patients.

Active Patients. For active patients, a random sampling can be approximated by simply giving a packet to every patient who arrives for an appointment in a given period—five hours, for instance, or five days, depending on the volume of your practice. (For a group practice, it is important to adjust the survey period so that it includes the days of the week on which each practitioner sees patients.) When patients are greeted upon arriving for an office visit, each can be asked to complete a patient-care survey, then given a packet with the explanatory letter and the questionnaire. That will give them the opportunity to complete the survey while they wait, and should ensure a higher rate of return than would be likely with a take-home survey.

The sample letter on the next page asks patients to place their completed survey in a box at the front desk. Before the survey begins, a clearly marked box must be placed at or near the front desk. The box should be big enough to hold all of the questionnaires that will be collected during the survey period.

Consider extending the survey period, if too few responses are obtained. About twenty-four responses per doctor is a good number.

Dear patient,

Thank you so much for participating in our anonymous survey. As we've already told you, we want to know how you feel about your experiences in our office. We are ready to hear whatever you have to say!

We promise to respectfully read and consider all comments, positive as well as negative, because of our commitment to giving all our patients the very best of care.

After completing this questionnaire, please deposit it in the box at the front desk before you leave.

Thank you very much for your assistance.

Sampling of Inactive Patients. This is a little more complicated than surveying the active patients, and involves a two-way mailing. It therefore should be started first, so that the two surveys can be more or less simultaneous.

The survey list can be compiled by taking every third name, say, from a list of patients whose last visit was three to six months ago—if that's what you consider an inactive patient. Or three to six weeks, or years, depending on the nature of your practice. You know how long a patient has to have been gone to be considered an ex-patient. This is a good job to give to someone who is new to the office and cannot be tempted to exclude or include particular patients. For each doctor, compile a survey list of at least 100 randomly selected inactive patients, then divide it in two. Send out fifty questionnaires in an initial mailing, reserving the other fifty names in case the response is insufficient. Remember, you want at least twenty-four responses per doctor.

The sample letter says that a stamped, addressed envelope is enclosed, which the patient can use to return the completed questionnaire to your office. Enclosing such an envelope will dramatically increase your response rate, saving you the cost of copying more letters and questionnaires, stuffing more envelopes, and paying the postage for another mailing.

Remember, while this survey is intended to detect possible problems in the way your office handles patients, it also is an opportunity to renew contact with patients whom you have not seen in a while. Many may not think of themselves as ex-patients, so be careful not to call them that—or to let them know that you consider them ex-patients. It is more productive to think of them as possible future patients or sources of possible referrals.

The letter below has been designed to encourage people to think of themselves as patients; to minimize any embarrassment about having missed a routine checkup or two, if they just haven't gotten around to scheduling an appointment; and to convince those who left because they were dissatisfied that your office may be ready to hear about and address the problem that drove them away.

Dear patient,

It's been a while since we've seen you, so you may not have heard that we have embarked upon a new program of quality assurance and evaluation. We want to ensure that we will provide an optimal environment for healing—and we are ready to hear whatever you have to say!

We hope you will agree to participate with us in this project by taking just a few minutes to fill out the enclosed anonymous survey.

We promise to respectfully read and consider all comments, positive as well as negative, because of our commitment to giving all our patients the very best of care.

After completing this questionnaire, please return it in the enclosed stamped, self-addressed envelope.

Thank you very much for your assistance. And please let us know when we can again be of service to you, your family, or your friends.

PATIENT EVALUATION QUESTIONNAIRE

What can we do to serve you better?

1. Are you generally satisfied with your experience at our office?
COMMENTS:

2. Are you greeted promptly and appropriately when you arrive?
COMMENTS:

3. Are you comfortable with the way we communicate with you? Are your questions answered, and is everything explained to your satisfaction?
COMMENTS:

4. Are you comfortable with the way all treatments and examinations are performed? With the way all office procedures are performed?
COMMENTS:

5. Would you send a family member or a friend to see us?
COMMENTS:

6. Is there anyone, or any type of person, whom you would not be comfortable sending to this office?
COMMENTS:

7. Have you heard any negative comments about our office? How can we ensure that everyone is satisfied with the care we provide?
COMMENTS:

8. Are you the same gender as your doctor (that is, male or female)? Do you prefer a doctor of the same gender?
COMMENTS:

9. Would you recommend any changes in our office procedures? In the way our staff deals with patients?
COMMENTS:

10. Have we always been sensitive to your needs?
COMMENTS:

11. What improvements would you recommend, to help us provide even better care?
COMMENTS:

If you don't mind, it might help us to know:
your gender: female   male
your age: 10-20   21-30   31-40   41-50   51-60   61-70   71-80   81 or older

PUTTING IT ALL TOGETHER

Congratulations! You've done well to get this far. Now that you've gotten all the questionnaires back, it's time to tabulate the results.

To paraphrase Abraham Lincoln's famous words to a caller at the White House: It is true that you may please all the people some of the time; you can even please some of the people all of the time; but you can't please all of the people all of the time.[1]

No matter how good a practitioner you are, there will be negative responses; be prepared. If you didn't get any negative responses, we want to meet you. But remember, positive comments are as important as negative comments. Both can help you to learn what is wrong and what is right about the way your practice operates. And don't just concentrate on what may be wrong with your practice. Praise your staff and yourself for all the things that are working.

Special Instructions

For the Doctor Self-Evaluation. Have at least one other person look over the DSE questionnaire, so that you can get another point of view. If you are working with a buddy or a supervisor, give him or her a copy of your completed questionnaire to review.

For the Staff Evaluation. Staff comments may be the most difficult to face, because they come from people you work with every day. And if any of the comments are very negative, you might find it difficult not to retaliate, no matter what you may have promised. If possible, therefore, have someone else do the initial review of Part I of the Staff Evaluation Questionnaire—the part that asks the staff for comments about you and the way you practice—and just give you the tabulated results. Knowing that you will not see the actual questionnaires and will not know who made which comments also may encourage your staff to give answers that are more honest and complete.

Option 1: Have a staff member tabulate the results, according to the instructions below, then give the results to you.

Option 2: Hire someone—even a temporary clerical worker—to tabulate the results.

Option 3: If you are working with a buddy or supervisor, consider having him or her review and tabulate the staff questionnaires. When you meet, he or she will sum up the staff's comments as well as the results of the Buddy/Supervisor questionnaire.

Option 4: Review and tabulate the staff questionnaires yourself, but beware of potential pitfalls. Staff members may be less than forthcoming. They may say only nice things. Or, if someone has a gripe, he or she may say only negative things. Read between the lines. And please *do not even attempt this* if you are very sensitive, have a bad temper, tend to hold a grudge, or have a hard time accepting criticism.

For the Patient Questionnaires. Consider having someone else do the initial work of tabulating the results. This is likely to be time-consuming and may be emotionally draining.

Option 1: Have a member of your staff tabulate the results and give them to you.

Option 2: Hire someone—even a temporary clerical worker—to tabulate the results.

Option 3: If you are working with a buddy or supervisor, have your staff or your temporary worker tabulate the results and give them to the buddy or supervisor.

Option 4: If you are working with a buddy or supervisor, have the buddy/supervisor review and tabulate the results.

Option 5: Review and tabulate the questionnaires yourself.

For the Buddy/Supervisor Questionnaire. No options here! The initial analysis of these questionnaires should be performed by the buddy or supervisor. After the buddy or supervisor has had time to review and organize his or her responses, and to decide how to present the comments and suggestions, the two of you should schedule a meeting—after hours or on a day off—at which you can discuss the findings.

Tabulating the Practice Evaluation Questionnaires

Prepare Tally Forms. Begin by preparing forms on which to tally the responses. The simplest way is to take a pad of lined paper, and label a separate sheet with each of the following categories.

- doctor attributes
- doctor attitudes
- doctor behaviors
- doctor skills
- staff attitudes
- staff behaviors
- staff skills
- office environment
- office procedures

One clearly labeled set of forms will be needed for the Doctor Self-Examination; another, for the Staff Evaluation; another, for the Patient Evaluation; and yet another for the Buddy/Supervisor Evaluation, if that is being performed (preliminary analysis of this questionnaire will be performed by the buddy or supervisor, but having the results presented on similar forms will make for easier comparisons later). You may need to make additional copies of some of these forms if there are many comments or if you have a large staff.

Keeping track separately of the comments from the questionnaires for the doctor, staff, patients, and buddy/supervisor, if applicable, will make it easier to compare the doctor's point of view with the staff's and patients'. And that, in turn, will make it easier to identify problems and figure out how to solve them.

A narrow column at the left of each sheet—two columns, in the case of patient responses, unless separate forms are being used for active patients and inactive patients—will be used to keep track of how many people gave the same response. The rest of each line will be used to report the responses themselves. (For an abbreviated example, see page 154).

Getting Started. Tally one sort of questionnaire at a time, and one survey form at a time. Consider tallying all comments, positive or negative, for a more complete view of the weak points and the strong points of your practice. If you choose to tally only the negative comments, you will need to watch very carefully at this stage for "sugar-coated criticisms" or "damning with faint praise." Some things to watch for:

- Sugar-coated criticisms. Some comments may be generally positive, maybe overly so, yet may hint that something needs work. To avoid missing these hidden hints, be sure to read every positive comment carefully.
- Critical responses. If someone is willing to express criticism, be grateful for that. Pay close attention to any and all criticisms, especially those that point to being inappropriate in terms of gender, sexuality and touch issues.
- Praise—especially if it is particularly glowing or faint. If it's glowing, don't let it go to your head—at least not right away. Read carefully between the lines to see if there is any shred of dissatisfaction, or hints that you could do something better. And think about this: Is any comment *too* positive? Could that indicate a possible infatuation? Just what is being praised? What *isn't* this person praising?
- Blaming the patient (this applies mostly to staff responses). Comments about patients being loud, whiny, obnoxious, demanding, or complaining probably indicate problems with the way your staff feels about, greets, or serves your patients.
- Any indication, even in jest, of a lack of respect.
- Any indication, even a hint, that someone is made uncomfortable by your attitudes or behaviors, or anyone else's. Each such comment reflects a potential problem.

As you come to each comment on the first questionnaire, decide which category is most appropriate, and copy the comment onto the corresponding analysis sheet. Place a single mark—"1"—in front of the comment, in the analysis sheet's left column, to indicate that one such comment has been received.

Some questionnaires are likely to include many comments, some very few. Be sure to copy every comment before moving on to the next survey form.

Keeping Track of Extreme Comments. If any of the survey responses include comments that are very negative, angry, very positive, have sexual overtones, seem to be complaints about touch and intimacy, or are just plain confusing, include them in your tally. But also draw a red circle around every such comment. When you are done tallying the comments from such a questionnaire, set it aside in a separate pile, with others that also had extreme comments, so you can look at them again later, after everything has been tabulated.

Keeping Your Cool. If you are tallying the results yourself, don't try to ignore your emotions. If you find yourself having strong feelings, pay attention to how you feel; this may be valuable information. But do try to keep your emotions in check. If you become overwrought, please take a break.

Dealing with Repeated Comments. When you come to a response that repeats an earlier comment, or is almost the same, don't write the comment down again. Just place another "1" in front of the comment you already have copied. Keep doing this until you are done with all of the questionnaires. At the end, count all of the "1s" in front of each comment, and write down the total.

| No. of Responses | | *SAMPLE ANSWERS, PATIENT QUESTIONNAIRES* |
active	inactive	Patient Comments
Doctor Behavior		
1	1111(4)	I don't like the way the doctor touches me
111 (3)	111 (3)	The doctor's hands are always so cold
11(4)	1111(4)	The doctor never explains what I'm supposed to do
11 (2)		I wish the doctor would stop hugging me
1		The doctor is so sexy—is she single? (This could fit into another category.)
Doctor Attitudes		
		The doctor is always cold
		The doctor is so friendly; maybe too friendly
		The doctor always uses words I don't understand
		The doctor always rushes, and has no time for me
		The doctor is impatient when I try to ask questions
Doctor Skills		
		The doctor's touch is very rough
		The doctor never hurts me
		The doctor is always so gentle
		The doctor examines my body but ignores ME; it's like I'm not even there
Doctor Attributes (looks, gender, marital status, sexual orientation)		
		The doctor is gorgeous; is he single?
		I'd rather not have to see a lady doctor

No. of Responses		SAMPLE ANSWERS, PATIENT QUESTIONNAIRES
active	inactive	Patient Comments (continued)
		Staff Behavior
		They keep me standing at the front desk forever, even when I'm in pain
		I never know when I'm done and can get dressed
		I never know who will walk in on me next
		Staff Attitudes
		The people at the front desk are rude
		The staff acts as if everyone is a bother
		I like the way the receptionist flirts with me
		Staff Skills
		I get cut off every time they put me on hold
		That girl at the front desk is sweet, but she doesn't seem to know what she's doing
		Office Environment
		The office is always cold
		The scale is in the hall where everyone can see
		You can hear everything; there's no privacy
		Those gowns don't cover anything
		There's no place to put my things when I undress
		Office Procedures/Routines
		Why don't they ever call me back?
		I have to wait forever for appointments
		I don't like waiting in that little room for so long

Evaluating the Severity of Problems

To determine how great a risk a problem represents, ask yourself: If a patient were to bring this type of problem forward before a court of law, would you find yourself having a serious problem?

Highest Risk Problems. Very high risk problems might be those that meet the definition of sexual violation that has been proposed in Ontario, Canada (for a fuller description, see page 106). These are problems that are illegal, unethical, and damaging to patients. They include: Sexual acts, including oral, vaginal and anal intercourse; exams of breasts, genitals and/or the rectal area that are not appropriate, or that are performed without full, informed consent; masturbation by either the patient or physician in the presence of the other.

High Risk Problems. High risk problems may involve boundary violations, such as those that meet the definition of sexual impropriety that has been proposed in Ontario (see page 106). These problems are likely to be illegal, unethical, and damaging to patients. They include: Seductive gestures or communication, comments about sexual fantasies, inappropriate comments about sexual parts, kissing patients, fondling patients, dating patients.

Lower Risk Problems. Lower risk problems may involve blurred or unclear boundaries; a lack of respect for a patient, or for patients in general; a lack of touching skills; a lack of skill in dealing with sexuality issues in practice; a lack of understanding of the effect of gender and power on doctor/patient communication; a failure to obtain full, informed consent for every procedure; a failure to listen to the patient and respect his or her wishes; a lack of communication skills. While lower risk problems are not the most serious, they still may suffice to drive away patients or put your practice in legal jeopardy. In addition, one or more lower risk problems may indicate, add up to, or even create a high risk problem.

Taking a Closer Look

With assistance, if necessary, determine which comments indicate a possible highest-risk or high-risk problem; whether the problem involves behaviors or attitudes; and who that problem involves—you, the staff, or both.

Examples of "High-Risk" Comments.

Comments That Might Indicate . . .

Problem Behaviors	Problem Attitudes
I wonder whether I've been touched in inappropriate ways.	The doctor seems attracted to me—is he available?
I feel uncomfortable when I run into the doctor outside the office.	I wonder why the doctor seems so interested in my sex life.
I wish they would tell me what they're doing, before they start.	I feel powerless with the doctor. He's in control of me.
The doctor tells me his personal problems. I don't know if it's okay.	I know the doctor is going through a crisis. I'm trying to help.
I don't think the doctor should be calling me just to talk.	I always seem to end up comforting the doctor. Isn't that his job?
I wish the doctor would stop inviting me to social events.	I sometimes wonder whether something sexual is going on.

Examples of "Lower Risk" Comments.

Comments That Might Indicate Possible . . .

Problem Behaviors	Problem Attitudes
The doctor's touch isn't comfortable.	I feel the doctor doesn't understand what I need.
The doctor always seems so rushed.	
I don't like it when the doctor asks to hug me.	Sometimes I think the doctor doesn't really see who I am.
Goodbye hugs last too long with the doctor.	I really look up to the doctor; he's like an idol to me.
The doctor seems to be doing so much for me.	I rely on the doctor a lot.
I really appreciate the way you folks are always willing to bend the rules.	It's a great office, but I feel uncomfortable sometimes.
Why is the wait always so long?	I feel awkward being alone in the office with the doctor.

How do you feel about each comment? Are you defensive, angry or resentful? Are you unable to comprehend—is your response, "I can't believe that someone could say something like that about me"?

What does each comment indicate about you or about the staff? What changes might be called for? (When you have decided what changes need to be made right away, turn to the next chapter, "Making Changes.")

If there were any comments that had been circled in red and set aside for later review—especially ones involving gender, sexuality or touch, or indicating a lack of respect—look at them now, too. (See Possible Warning Signs, page 136.) You might want to look all of these over with a friend or colleague, one comment at a time.

Remember, even the lower risk problems have a detrimental effect on your practice. They may be related to, or indicate a vulnerability to, more serious problems. And many lower risk problems can offend patients and make them feel uncomfortable; they reduce referrals, and may cause patients to leave and not come back.

Looking for Patterns. Ask yourself: Am I a power figure? Do I have a need to be right? Do I treat my patients fairly? Do I allow my patients to tell me what they want?

- There may be a pattern of problems with touch or communication.
- Looking more deeply, you may find that this pattern indicates problems with power and a lack of respectful care, or problems with the obtaining of patient consent.
- Sexually inappropriate comments or behavior may indicate that a person lacks awareness about what is appropriate, or lacks awareness of his or her own sexuality.
- A pattern of risky behavior may hint at a personal or professional crisis that may be affecting the practice.
- There may be a pattern of difficulties with patients of a particular gender, which

might indicate a problem with attitudes toward that gender or a need to learn to better understand that gender's communication style.

- There may be a pattern of problems with patients of a particular age group or socioeconomic class; this might indicate problems with handling power or a lack of flexibility and range in a person's communication style.

COMPARING THE RFA AND PRACTICE EVALUATIONS

Because the Risk-Factor Analysis and the Practice Evaluation Questionnaires do not do exactly the same things, it is entirely possible to have a high-risk score on one and a low-risk score on the other. The Practice Evaluation Questionnaires emphasize external factors: the methods, skills and behaviors you bring to your practice. The RFA emphasizes internal factors: the attitudes and beliefs you bring to your practice, and your current level of stress.

If both your RFA and the Practice Evaluation Questionnaires—not only your self-evaluation but also the staff and patient surveys—uncover few problems with the way you practice, then congratulations! You and your patients probably are at very low risk, and chances are, you are very popular and have a thriving practice. Keep up the good work.

If your RFA indicates possible problems, but in the Practice Evaluation Questionnaires you come out smelling like a rose, then it is likely that you are doing a good job of protecting your patients and yourself, but that you either have weaknesses that ought to be addressed or are going through a stressful period that increases your vulnerability.

Questions to Consider

Did you complete only the self-evaluation questionnaire? If so, it is possible there are problems in your practice of which you are not aware. Everybody has blind spots. That is why the staff and patient questionnaires are so important.

Were you surprised by any of the answers that were given by your patients and staff in the Practice Evaluation Questionnaires? If your RFA results were good, but the other questionnaires indicate a high level of problems in the office, you'll need to look more closely at the way you relate to your patients and staff.

In their questionnaires, did your patients or staff indicate that they thought your attitudes were a problem or a potential problem? If so, you might have more than procedural difficulties to resolve. You might want to reexamine Chapter 4, "Explorations and Applications."

Did the RFA and the Practice Evaluation Questionnaires both indicate problems? Then it's time for some serious work. It also is time to seriously consider some outside supervision, both to help you make the necessary changes and to help keep you out of trouble while you do. This could be provided by a professional supervisor, or it could be provided by a carefully selected "buddy"—someone who you trust and respect, but who does *not* share the attitudes and behaviors that you have identified as a problem.

DECIDING WHAT TO CHANGE

Figure Out What to Change

Determine what changes need to be made by the doctor, by the staff, and in the office. (See the next chapter, "Making Changes.")

It is important to take immediate action on any highest risk or high risk problems you may have identified, even if a complete fix will take some time. The lower risk problems also should be promptly addressed. If you didn't identify any, congratulations! In that case, you can afford to spend some time mulling the results of the Safe Practice Assessment before deciding how you would like to modify your practice.

Don't Panic

Some changes might be very easy to make, while others may require a long-term commitment. Sometimes, just being aware of what you are doing and how it is being perceived can make all the difference.

Making changes in habits that are deeply ingrained can be difficult. This is especially the case when we attempt to break old habits or try to change unconscious patterns. A little assistance may be in order. This help could be from a buddy or supervisor, or from a counselor or psychotherapist.

Figure Out How to Change

Now that you have an understanding of how your practice looks from a patient's point of view, it's time to decide what to do about it. A brainstorming session can be a good place to start.

Have everyone in the office get together and make a list of all the patient suggestions you received—even the ones that are silly or insulting. Use a very large pad and have one person be the scribe (someone with good handwriting) and write down every one of the suggestions. Even the silly ones may have a shred of brilliance.

Then, discuss ways in which your practice can correct each problem the survey has revealed. Don't just focus on the problem areas that were highlighted by the questionnaires; also discuss how you could expand upon the things you are already doing well. Again, write everything down. If some of the solutions seem pretty wacky, that's fine. You won't actually use them all.

Next, get serious. Sort through all those ideas, and decide what your office actually could do, and should do, to make things run more smoothly. Some changes you might want to make right away; others might take longer to incorporate into your practice.

Don't Forget the Follow-Up

Follow-through is very important. Let your patients know what you are doing with their suggestions. If you just file away their questionnaires, that will expose your lack of commitment to making improvements in your practice, as you told your patients you would do. Instead, keep them involved. Let them know that you care what they think, and that you really do value their opinions.

Consider posting a list of some of the suggestions you received, highlighting the ones you intend to use, and explaining when and how they will be implemented. A one-page office newsletter could be used to keep patients up-to-date on the changes you have made, and ones you plan to make. If your practice doesn't already have comment cards or a suggestion box in the waiting room, this is a good time to start.

Keep records. Six months or a year from now, take the time to go over the survey results again. What has changed? What hasn't? Are there problems that still need to be addressed? Are there things that used to be standard practice that now, you wouldn't even consider doing that way?

NOTE

1. The word that President Lincoln actually used was "fool," not "please." He was referring to the fragility of trust, and explaining why he believed that honesty was always the best policy.

— *14* —

Making Changes

It isn't easy to change, but you've already taken the hardest step: acknowledging that change is necessary. Here is a four-step process that can be help you to make whatever changes are indicated:[1]

1. Determine the exact nature of your problem—who, where, when, why.
2. Find a solution.
3. Put the solution into action.
4. Assess the efficacy of your action step(s).

DIAGNOSING THE PROBLEM

Problems Involving Touch

Recognition. Touch, quality of touch, or use of touch was mentioned as a problem. Patients may have complained about roughness, about being tickled (if the tickling was not intentional, this may indicate too light or unsteady a touch), about accidental touch during or after a procedure.

Hints for Correction. Read Chapter 3, "Touch," and study Chapter 11, the "Safe Touch Protocol."

Problems Involving Consent

Recognition. Patients may have mentioned that they were not asked about something, that a procedure was not explained, that they did not understand the explanation, that their questions were not answered, that exams or procedures were done before they were ready, that they were startled, that their refusal for a procedure to be performed was ignored, that a procedure was not terminated when consent was withdrawn.

Hints for Correction. Read over Chapter 11, the "Safe Touch Protocol," especially the part regarding obtaining consent.

Problems Involving Communication

Recognition. There would have had to have been a mention of communication, but it might have been oblique: Perhaps patients said that they were interrupted, that the visit was terminated before they were ready, that they did not know when the visit was over, that they did not know whether or how much to disrobe, that they did not know when to get dressed, that the practitioners did not seem to listen when they stated their priorities, that their problem was never diagnosed, that they didn't understand the diagnosis, that they didn't understand treatment instructions, or that they were treated rudely. (See also the section below on Problems Involving Power or Respect.)

Hints for Correction. First, it is necessary to determine what is not being communicated, and by whom, or where communication is breaking down. Only then can you make attempts to alter those specific things. Whatever the problem is, these steps will help to alleviate it:

- Develop better listening and communication skills—verbal and nonverbal.
- Become an expert in communication.

For hints on dealing with specific communication problems, consult Chapter 4, "Explorations and Applications."

Problems Involving Power or Respect

Recognition. The words "respect" or "power" may not be used; instead, look for words that give a hint of this sort of thing. Key words and phrases might include: the doctor/nurse/staff is rude; when I ask questions, the doctor/nurse/staff acts as if it's a nuisance; they don't answer my questions; when they answer my questions, they talk fast and use big words, and I never know what they said; I don't feel included; I can't get a word in edgewise; the doctor doesn't even care what I think; the doctor/nurse/staff just tells me what to do; the doctor/nurse/staff never even tells me what is going to be done (note: this indicates that your practice may need to pay more attention to the legal and ethical issue of informed consent); they always keep me waiting; why do they have me undress, just to sit in that tiny room alone?; they make me walk across the office half-naked; they walk in on me when I'm changing; the office is so cold—it's fine for the doctor, he's wearing lots of clothes, but I always freeze.

Hints for Correction. The key is to see yourself not as a superior but as an equal—one who happens to have skills and knowledge that the patient probably does not. Remember that the patient's time and the patient's comfort are as valuable as your own, that the patient's opinions must be honored. Try to be a good host.

- Share information: Try to see yourself as a teacher, rather than as a parent or a doctor. Remember, patients are more likely to follow instructions that they understand.

- Don't leave patients in the dark: When a patient is sent somewhere, or left somewhere, be sure the patient knows what will happen next and roughly how long he or she will have to wait. If the situation changes, keep the patient informed.
- Respect patients' privacy: Hold private discussions in private places. Keep equipment used by gowned patients in a private place; if patients often are moved around while gowned, take that into consideration when deciding what gowns to order.
- Respect patients' schedules: This is one of patients' biggest gripes about doctors. If patients often have to wait for their appointment, is there some way your practice could minimize waiting times? If patients often wait for long periods in the exam rooms, is there some way that time can be minimized?
- Respect patients' comfort: Remember, the patient probably is immobile, while you are active. Either keep the office at a comfortable temperature for gowned patients, and dress more lightly yourself, or provide robes or blankets.

For additional hints on power and respect, see Chapter 9, "The Doctor Role."

Problems Involving Attractions

Recognition. Patients are attracted to you; you are attracted to patients; patients are attracted to a staff member; a staff member is attracted to patients; a staff member is attracted to you; you are attracted to a staff member.

If such a dynamic is present, it takes the focus off caring for patients. Patients probably are being harmed. The practice could be harmed.

Hints for Correction. If there's a problem with patients being attracted to you, or you being attracted to patients, or with a staff attraction, something needs to be done. Don't ignore the situation.

- Address the problem immediately, for the patient and yourself.
- Get help if necessary.
- Figure out what happened and why, and do whatever is necessary to keep it from happening again.

For additional hints, read Chapter 15, "Defusing Sexual Attractions."

Problems Involving Boundaries

Recognition. Look for any of these key words, phrases, or concepts in the comments:

- "Inappropriate."
- Patient felt "strange" or "uncomfortable" or "uneasy."
- Someone—patient, staff, supervisor, or buddy—questions the need for a specific procedure, or questions the way it was performed.
- Concerns about professionalism are raised.
- Difficulty dealing with doctor or staff behavior is mentioned.

• Doctor or staff get "too personal."

Hints for Correction. See Chapter 11, the "Safe Touch Protocol," and Chapter 12, the "Safe Practice Strategies." Re-read the discussion of professional boundaries in Chapter 8, "Boundaries and Consent." Pay particular attention to:

• Awareness of the vulnerability of both patient and doctor.
• Sensitivity to the needs of patients.
• Awareness of the power of the doctor role.

These are only general guidelines for use in making those changes that may have been highlighted by the Safe Practice Analysis. We all know that the more deeply entrenched the attitude and behavior are, the more difficult it is to change them. But it's worth it.

WHEN OTHERS SAY YOU HAVE A PROBLEM

Accepting the Need for Change
When faced with the challenge of making changes, there are two ways in which one might respond.

You Do Not Accept that You Need to Make Changes. This position makes improvement difficult, but not impossible.

If you are unable to comprehend what others are trying to tell you, then you need to see a therapy professional, your buddy, your supervisor, or a colleague whom you trust and respect. That person may be able to help you with this.

If you are unwilling to do that and insist that you are the one who's right, be aware that you may be at risk. You are taking a chance in continuing to practice as you are. Remember, right or wrong, what you are doing is generating complaints or concern. Consider making changes to improve patient satisfaction.

Making changes may be difficult. But, the consequences of not changing could be great.

You Accept that Change Is Indicated. Congratulations on your willingness and openness. This makes it easier, but not necessarily easy, to make the indicated adjustments. It will be worth the effort to ensure a safe and comfortable environment for your patients and yourself.

Addressing Concerns Raised by Staff

High-Risk Problems. If you learn that a staff member believes you have a high risk problem, take these steps:

• Schedule a private meeting with the staff.
• Let them know you appreciate their feedback and honesty.

- If you have difficulty accepting their comments or criticisms, ask for specific examples. Ask them to point it out to you shortly after you've done it again.
- If you agree with the concerns they have raised, let them know. Ask for their assistance in pointing out the problem behavior when it arises.
- Explain that you've done lots of self-evaluating, and are trying to improve the way you practice.
- Be sure to thank and praise the staff for their willingness to help you.
- When staff members take the time to point things out to you, thank them.
- Make any necessary changes, as you can.
- Let the staff know when and how you are making changes.

Lower-Risk Problems. When staff comments indicate the presence of a lower-risk problem, take these steps:

- Call a staff meeting to go over all material you've uncovered.
- Praise the staff members for their honesty.
- Point out where you agree and where you disagree with their assessment. Ask for specific examples. Ask them to point out the problem when it happens.
- Thank them for their help.
- Let them know how much you want to change—but only if that's true.
- Let them know when and how you are making changes.

Addressing Concerns Raised by Patients
Go through the processing questions below. Then go to the action steps listed later in this chapter, under Making Changes in Doctor Behaviors.

Processing Questions.
- Was the handling of any one procedure, or type of procedure, the target of a great deal of praise or criticism?
- Were there many comments, positive or negative, about one staff member or practitioner?
- What kind of differences can you find in the responses of active versus inactive patients?
- Is there some common complaint?
- Is there some kind of person (old/young, male/female) who seems to be happiest or unhappiest with you or your practice?
- What can you tell about the individuals responding? Can you determine whether they are a professional or not? who responded the most? the least?
- Can you tell whether they are conservative or liberal? Anything else?
- What blind spots might you or your practice have?
- In what areas could it stand to be improved?
- What is your practice doing that doesn't seem to work? That does?

MAKING CHANGES

Making Changes in Doctor Behaviors

There are three steps to take. First, ask yourself processing questions. Second, take action. Remember, even if a problem seems to be overwhelming, be aware that taking baby steps in the right direction can have profound and positive effects. Third, review the action with processing questions. All three can be done alone or with assistance.

Remember, don't expect miracles overnight. Accepting the need for change is half the battle, and that alone may be enough to bring some progress, but lasting change takes time.

Processing Questions.
- Where does this belief/behavior comes from?
- Who in your life believes/behaves that way?
- What are the benefits to believing/behaving this way?
- Do you pay a price for such a belief/behavior? If so, what is it?
- What small change can you make in this belief/behavior that doesn't feel too abrupt?
- How does this belief/behavior affect your relationships with patients?
- After the change, what will your new relationship with patients be like?

Actions.
- Observe your attitudes, beliefs, and behavior as you work.
- Ask for help—get impressions, feelings and thoughts from staff, patients, friends, colleagues, supervisor, or buddy as you focus on making changes.
- Write yourself notes, to remind yourself to think/behave differently. Place these notes where you will see them.
- Make an effort to pay attention to how your beliefs affect you, your patients and staff. Watch everyone you interact with closely.
- Pay attention to the way you communicate. Ask others to do so also. It contains clues about beliefs and behaviors, as well as communication skills and styles.
- Be the recipient of that belief or behavior—put yourself in the patient's shoes. Or, ask someone to behave that way toward you.
- Create an affirmation. Use it.
- Keep a journal of the difference your efforts are making and how you're doing.
- When you notice that you have done well, give yourself lots of compliments.

Processing Questions.
- Has what I have done differently made a difference in how patients respond to me?
- If yes, what has changed?
- Do I feel any different when I behave differently? How so?
- If I did it alone, was I able to make those changes?
- If I got help, was it helpful? Did it make me defensive in some way?

Making Changes in Staff Behavior

Remember that for staff members, too, accepting the need for change is the first, most difficult step in this process. Care and respect are needed in initial discussions of staff behavior problems, or a hostile environment may be created.

Dealing with High-Risk Staff Problems.

Such problems might include flirting with patients, walking in on patients when they are naked or half-dressed, or touching patients inappropriately.

- Schedule a private meeting with the staff member.
- Use the sandwich approach: Give praise first, then criticism, and finish with praise.
- Motivate the staff member: Explain that making this change is critical for the practice and for his or her future there.
- Try to involve the staff member in setting reasonable goals; be sure that the goals are clear, and that the staff member understands what is expected of him or her.
- Take and keep good notes of this meeting and all related interactions, both to track progress and for your own protection.
- Have a follow-up meeting. If no change has yet been made, reemphasize the importance of change and tell the staff member you will review the situation again within about a week.
- At that time, if there has been no progress since the second meeting, discharge this employee (consider seeking legal counsel on how to do this appropriately).

Dealing with Lower-Risk Staff Problems.

Such problems might include a staff member who has an abrupt touch, or who is considered rude.

- Schedule a private meeting with this staff member.
- Use the sandwich approach: Give praise first, then a criticism, and follow up with praise.
- Try to involve the staff member in setting reasonable goals; be sure that the goals are clear, and that the staff member understands what is expected of him or her.
- Motivate the staff member: Explain the importance of the change that is needed. Point out another member of the staff who well what this person does poorly. Praise the other staff member.
- Praise the staff member who does it correctly in front of everyone.
- Have a follow-up meeting. Praise any improvement; review and adjust goals together with the staff member. Praise the staff member in front of everyone.
- If there has been no change, try working on the problem together with this person, or asking another staff member to help.
- If there still is no change, consider assigning this person to do other work, if he or she has other skills.
- Make and keep good notes at the initial and follow-up meetings, both to track progress and for your own protection.

Don't Lose Your Perspective

Don't Expect Miracles. Half the progress comes just from knowing that change is necessary—but lasting changes aren't accomplished overnight.

Seek Help. Seek the assistance of your staff. Consider turning to a buddy, a supervisor, or a therapist.

Don't Panic. Some changes might be very easy to make, while others may require a long-term commitment. Sometimes, just an awareness of what we're doing can make all the difference. Making changes in attitudes or behaviors that are deeply ingrained is difficult. This is especially the case when attempting to break longstanding habits or try to change patterns of which one may not be consciously aware.

Reward Progress. When you notice that you have done well, give yourself lots of compliments and maybe a special treat. Likewise, don't forget to reward improvements by your staff.

WHEN PROBLEMS INVOLVE A BELIEF SYSTEM

If your beliefs or behaviors do not negatively affect your practice and your patients, then there is no problem. But, that is not a determination a person can make for himself or herself.

It is for this reason that the Safe Practice Analysis was created. From the results of the Practice Analysis, you will undoubtedly have learned what needs to change. And, from having read this book, we hope you will have gained some insights and gotten some ideas about how you might alter your ways of doing things. Now it's time to apply what you've learned.

We've divided these practical applications into a few categories:

It's important to understand your beliefs. Do you openly voice them? Are you secretive about them? Even if you don't voice them, do your patients pick up on them?

If your beliefs are extreme or unpopular, you'll need to take into account the effect that voicing or otherwise expressing such opinions could have on your practice. This doesn't mean that you should not be true to yourself. But it is rarely a good idea to use a practice as a platform. There is a point at which your expression of such beliefs could pose a problem for you or for your patients. If you are not careful, patients might become hesitant to volunteer information and might feel uncomfortable with you.

If you can be supportive of your patient's ideas and beliefs, rather than imposing your own, you will be doing a service to yourself and your patients.

NOTE

1. For those seeking more information on the process of behavioral change itself, University of Rhode Island professor James O. Prochaska's "Transtheoretical Model" provides an insightful and helpful analysis. An excellent reference is the comprehensive article "The Transtheoretical Model of Health Behavior Change" (Prochaska and Wayne F. Velicer, *American Journal of Health Promotion*, Sept. 1, 1997, 38), which describes his six stages of change and ten processes of change; discusses temptations and "decisional balance"; and includes examples of non-health-behavior applications.

— 15 —

Defusing Sexual Attractions

The sexual and loving dimensions of clinical practice can be dangerous for both practitioner and patient . . . if they remain silent, unnamed, and denied. Under these conditions, the potential for acting upon these feelings increases.

—Nancy A. Bridges,
"Meaning and Management of Attraction," 1994

There is, unfortunately, no magic formula for resolving the difficulties of a situation that brings sexuality into your practice. When an attraction occurs—whether it is yours, the patient's, or mutual—the situation is likely to demand a unique solution, because both you and your patient are unique.

Each profession has specific guidelines regarding nonprofessional relationships, particularly romantic ones. Be certain that you know what they are. Write down everything that transpires between you, in the patient's records. Consider seeking some sort of supervision or outside advice; there is no time when you will need it more.

When a sexual "situation" presents itself in your practice, the power is in your hands to safeguard the patient, as well as yourself. But you can do this only if you carefully monitor yourself, as well as the patient. "A stereotypical response of beginning clinicians is to ignore sexual feelings with and toward patients until they become unbearable."[1] Unfortunately, this course of action only increases the risk to both parties. Ignoring or repressing the problem will not make it go away. It will only remove it from rational consideration.

It is necessary—when sexual overtones intrude into the doctor/patient relationship—to tread a very thin line, remaining caring while becoming neither cold and distant nor too friendly. If you feel unable to do this, you should consider referring this patient to someone who can.

The best way to prepare for such encounters with patients is to attend training sessions that offer opportunities for role-playing. In such trainings, you will learn about the strategies and ideas that other practitioners have used, and you will construct your own. In this way, you will build important doctor/patient relationship skills.

Here are some possible ways to think about and deal with four possible scenarios. They are presented for you to use in preparing yourself for difficult situations; to refer to when such a situation arises in your practice; and to consider if you are asked to advise a colleague who is experiencing such difficulties. But these are merely an abstract guide—a virtual role-playing experience, if you will—and are no substitute for expert advice on your particular situation from a lawyer or trained supervisor.

YOU SUSPECT A PATIENT ATTRACTION

Discussion

You sense the patient is attracted to you, but the patient has not told you. You may be right. You may be wrong. You *must* be careful.

Ask yourself: What makes you suspect an attraction? Something the patient said? Something the patient did? Is it possible that you are projecting your own feelings onto the patient?

Guidelines

1. Do not ask patients whether they are attracted to you.

2. Do not tell a patient that you are picking this up from him or her.

3. You might begin to display pictures of your significant other around the office, or casually mention something the two of you recently did together.

4. If you don't have a significant other, if you are breaking up with your significant other, or if you have recently been through a break-up, do not share this information with the patient.

YOU ARE TOLD OF A PATIENT ATTRACTION

Discussion

If a patient tells you that he or she is attracted to you, start by asking yourself whether you could have had any responsibility for this attraction. Does this happen to you often? Are you attracted to this patient? Whether you are attracted or not, are you flattered by the attention? How flattered are you? Are you encouraging this patient? Do you often enjoy and perhaps encourage this sort of attention and admiration from your patients? How vital is such attention to you? A mentor or colleague could help you to sort through these questions.

Even if your attitude and behavior are not contributing to the problem, patients still may become attracted to you. This may be because you look like Mel Gibson or Sharon Stone—but if that is not the case, then the reason is likely to be that the role of doctor is so very powerful. (See Chapter 9, "The Doctor

Role'' for more information on the power of the role of doctors.) Another possible contributor is the traditional belief that doctors are a ''good catch.''

Guidelines

1. Whenever a patient expresses an interest in you, very gently tell him or her that you are not available. If you are married or in a relationship, then say so; if you are not, don't lie, just don't mention that you are single. Say that, in any case, you don't date patients. Thank the patient for telling you, and let him or her know you are honored by the interest.

Some doctors might even feel comfortable saying to the patient, ''That's great! That must mean you're feeling healthy and good about yourself, and that you're probably ready for someone special in your life.'' This offers the patient a way to save face, and also emphasizes the efficacy of your treatment.

2. From then on, be very sensitive and alert in your interactions with this patient. When you are caring for such patients, be careful about the way you look at, speak with, and touch them. Be extremely aware of your own attitude, and of all the messages you convey.

3. This might be a good time to seek the help of a mentor. If you do, then determine together whether this patient can continue to receive good care from you, or should be seen by someone else. Depending on the patient, you might consider letting him or her in on the decision-making as well.

4. Remember, the attraction that your patient feels may not be real; it may be an attraction to the doctor role, rather than to you. Doctors have a great deal of knowledge; have the power to cure or even save their patients; and usually adopt a professional demeanor that may make them seem to have it all together. In patients' eyes, you are bigger than life; as a result, they have difficulty acting normally around you. This phenomenon is called transference. Handling a patient's active transference requires tremendous sensitivity and caring, as well as good communication skills.

5. When a doctor gets caught up in a patient's transference (for instance, the patient sees you as bigger than life, and you believe it), the phenomenon is called countertransference. This is one of the pitfalls of practice: Believing ourselves to be what the patient sees us to be. If we encourage patients to see us as bigger than life, then we encourage and participate in the delusion.

YOU FEEL ATTRACTED TO A PATIENT

Discussion

Ask yourself: Does this happen often? What are the patients like, to whom you are attracted? Is there a pattern?

If you do not plan to act on this attention, pay particular attention to Guideline 1 below; if you have ever considered acting on this attraction, read Guidelines 2 and 3 over and over again.

Guidelines

1. It is vital to understand that the attraction you feel may not be real. The section on transference and countertransference, in Chapter 9, explains in greater detail how these two factors can affect the doctor and the patient. When a doctor feels attracted to a patient, it actually is very likely that he or she has fallen into a pattern that goes back to one or more past relationships. This is countertransference. The stronger the feelings, the more primal the connection tends to be. During a very intense attraction, it is easy to project onto the patient all sorts of feelings that one has had for others in the past. In other words, the feeling that one has fallen in love might actually be a delusion.

2. Denying the volatility of your feelings would be foolish. So would deciding not to seek help with sorting through those feelings. Such outside help could be provided by a supervisor, therapist, licensing board member, colleague or consultant. Ignoring the options that are available puts practitioners in a position to hurt their patients, to hurt themselves and to hurt their professions.

3. If you don't want help, and if you are determined to follow through with your attraction to a patient, at least consider what the effect might be on your patient. Are you really sure that a relationship with you would be beneficial for your patient? Many health professionals who have entered into sexual relationships with their patients have done so believing that such a relationship would be helpful for their patient. *The opposite has generally been true.* Patients, and the professionals to whom they turn after such an experience, almost unanimously agree that the patient was harmed.

THE ATTRACTION IS MUTUAL

Discussion

What if you and a patient are attracted to one another—and you both know it? It's one thing for a patient to be attracted to you; it's another, for you to be attracted to a patient; and it's yet another, when the feeling is mutual. But it's completely another to act on it. Re-read the scenarios above, for strategies for dealing with patient or doctor attractions. Then go on to the guidelines below.

Guidelines

1. Remember, this may just be a case of transference and countertransference, both of which can inspire very strong feelings. This is very difficult to determine alone, particularly since each of us has blind spots that impede clear vision. Consider supervision or psychotherapy; negotiating such difficult territory is easier and safer when one has a guide.

2. Consider consulting a lawyer.

3. If the two of you decide that you wish to date, you will need to take the following steps:

- you must dismiss this patient from your care;

- you must refrain from seeing this former patient in any capacity—personal or professional—for a certain period of time (Consult the guidelines for your profession. For marriage and family therapists, a two-year waiting period is required before a therapist and client may consider a romantic relationship; for pastoral counselors, it is never permissible to date a former client.);
- during the no-contact period, you and the former patient also must not speak to one another, or carry on a written correspondence;
- you must keep accurate records of exactly what occurs at each point in your relationship: what each of you said and did (you should be sure to do this, no matter what other course you decide to follow);
- you should consult with an outside professional (having consulted with someone during the decision-making process also would be helpful).

4. Be aware that if you and your patient have had a conversation about dating while he or she is still a patient, then your romantic or sexual relationship can considered to have begun while you were doctor and patient. This is true even if you then dismiss the patient, and the two of you don't start dating until later. If the relationship eventually turns sour, or if the patient later decides that it was inappropriate and harmful, the patient will be accurate in stating that the relationship began while you were doctor and patient. Try to avoid this potential pitfall.

5. Remember, if you do become romantically or sexually involved with a patient, you put your reputation and your livelihood at risk.

These guidelines may help in dealing with difficult situations. All attractions are complex and have the potential to affect those involved in many ways. Consider what this attraction brings out in you and what it means to you.

Be careful. Look within yourself. Get advice. Record everything. Remember, you bear the ultimate responsibility for whatever happens.

NOTE

1. Nancy A. Bridges, "Meaning and Management of Attraction: Neglected Areas of Psychotherapy Training and Practice," *Psychotherapy*, 31 (Fall 1994): 3, 425.

PART IV

Review

The sexual dimensions of clinical practice and relationships are dangerous when they are denied, projected, or otherwise disowned.

—Nancy A. Bridges,
"Meaning and Management
of Attraction," 1994

— *16* —

Six Factors for Safe Practice

THE TRUST FACTOR

Trust is a precious and fragile commodity that is hard to win yet easy to lose. And, as Abraham Lincoln put it, "If you once forfeit the confidence of your fellow citizens, you can never regain their respect and esteem." Once you have earned your patients' trust, do not violate it.

You have a fiduciary relationship with your patients, and that means that you have agreed to set aside your own interests in order to do what is best for them. You *must* put their comfort and welfare ahead of your wants and needs. Your personal agenda must be left on the other side of the closed door. This is the obligation of all health-care providers.

THE TOUCH FACTOR

Touch is a method of communication, capable of transmitting messages both conscious and unconscious, that is made no less powerful by Western society's tendency to overlook it. Touch is a necessary part of many doctor/patient interactions, but it should never be used carelessly.

Know yourself in relationship to touch. How do you feel about touch? How do you prepare yourself and your patients for touching? How is touching patients different from touching friends, lovers, or children?

Get feedback on your touch. How do people respond to the different kinds of touch you use? How do people describe your touch? What are its qualities? Is it comforting? Gentle? Healing? Strong? Rough? When you ask about how others perceive your touch, you may discover a need to practice certain touching skills or to make changes in the way you use touch in your practice.

Be aware of your patients' response to touch and near-touch. Though touch is a method of communication, it is one with many dialects. Attitudes toward touch and proximity vary widely from culture to culture, region to region, family to family, and even from individual to individual.

Always ask for permission before touching a patient. Explain what you will be doing and why. If the patient seems uncertain about what you plan to do, then explain it again, or ask the patient to describe what he or she expects to happen. Wait for consent; never assume consent. And if a patient withdraws consent at any point, stop.

Be very careful in your use of casual touch—that is, touch that is not a necessary part of a diagnostic or therapeutic procedure. This type of touch can easily be misused, or misinterpreted.

Be especially sensitive with those patients who you know have been sexually abused, or who you suspect may have been abused.

Be certain that your riskiest and most invasive procedures have been altered to create safety and comfort for all of your patients.

THE POWER FACTOR

The doctor/patient relationship is an unequal one. The doctor occupies a position of higher status and greater power, while the patient's position—weaker from the start—is often further weakened by the very problem that caused him or her to seek care. It is essential, therefore, to be sensitive to any behaviors on your part that could widen the gulf between doctor and patient. The following behaviors are ones that can exacerbate the imbalance between doctor and patient.

Hugging Patients

Hugging is taking a liberty with another person's body. Forcing such an intimacy on a patient is asking for trouble. If you still wish to hug your patients, always remember to ask first, and limit hugging to those patients who you are certain want to be hugged. Many patients may not feel comfortable with hugging, even among those who might say yes. Some may be so uncomfortable that they stop coming to you. Other patients may interpret the hugs you intended as a friendly gesture to mean that you are attracted to them.

For the most part, hugging between doctor and patient is best avoided. Yours is, after all, a professional relationship.

Hoarding Power

Insisting that patients use particular names or titles in referring to the doctor and staff can be part of an atmosphere of mutual respect. More often, however, it is a method of emphasizing and exaggerating the higher status of the care-givers, at the expense of the dignity of the cared-for. Habitually keeping patients waiting is another such method. So is having them march about the office half-naked. These common practices are signs and symptoms of a condescending attitude that can quell communication and extinguish rapport. They indicate that, consciously or not, you are using the power of the care-giver role to maintain a "one-up" position—of status and control—in the doctor/patient relationship.

Instead, try establishing an atmosphere in which respect and accommodation are mutual. There is nothing wrong with your requesting the use of certain preferred forms of address, for instance, so long as patients are permitted to do the same. Your patients' time and dignity should be valued as highly your own.

Hoarding Information

Using obscure professional jargon, without also translating that information into nontechnical terms, is holding onto knowledge rather than sharing it. This is another form of one-upmanship—of hoarding power. It may promote an image of learning and professional expertise, but it does not promote the health of the patient.

Instead, try tailoring your questions, answers, and advice to suit each patient's level of understanding. Give the patients time to ask questions; take the time to be sure they understand your answers.

THE DOCTOR FACTOR

Know Yourself

Be aware of your limits and weaknesses, both as a doctor and as a person. Seek guidance when you are feeling particularly vulnerable—whether because of a relationship problems, such as break-up or divorce, some other significant loss or emotional turmoil, loneliness, or an overactive libido. Ask a colleague or a supervisor/consultant/therapist for help. At potential crisis times like these, doctors are more likely to get themselves into difficulties.

Make every effort to treat all your patients equally. Ask yourself, "Would I be doing this if my patient were 55, fat, and balding, rather than an attractive 22-year-old aerobics instructor?" If you find yourself violating your own office policies, or giving a patient special consideration, beware. This is an early warning of possible problems.

Know your Patients

Recognize and respect *their* limits. Be certain that all procedures have been carefully thought out—and altered, where necessary—to maximize the safety and comfort of each of your patients. Minimize the possibility of misunderstanding by putting one of your friends or relatives through each of your normal procedures, having him or her play patient to your doctor. Have yourself put through your normal procedures, too, so you will better understand what your patients are experiencing.

Get a Second Opinion

Ask your patients and staff for feedback about your behavior—especially female patients and staff, who are likely to be more sensitive to nuances of touch and behavior. Have an anonymous questionnaire distributed randomly to some of your patients and staff. (Sample patient and staff questionnaires are presented in the "Safe Practice Analysis," Chapter 13.)

THE COMMUNICATION FACTOR

Fine-tune your communication skills so that your communication with patients is as clear, respectful, and patient-centered as possible. Before speaking, ask yourself, "How will what I am about to say affect this patient?"

When communicating about procedures that could create increased vulnerability for patients, be especially careful. Patients must be given the opportunity to consent to procedures, or to decline. And they must be given respect, regardless of what decision they make.

When speaking with patients, and when addressing them, be careful not to be patronizing. Avoid the use of "honey" and "dear"—some people find the use of these terms of endearment by a near-stranger to be demeaning and offensive—and remember that "girl" is best limited to female patients well under the age of 18.

Use compliments with care. They can be perfectly harmless, but they also can be misused or misinterpreted. Ask yourself, "Would this pass for a pickup line at a singles bar?" or "Would I feel comfortable saying this if the patient's significant other or a trained supervisor were in the room?" Especially avoid giving compliments while your hands are on a patient.

Let patients have their say. Remember the advice of Ernest Hemingway: "When people talk, listen completely. Most people never listen." You may be the expert on health-care, but the patient is the expert on his or her condition. Listening respectfully, without interrupting, takes only a few moments longer, permits more of that valuable information to emerge, and leaves the patient in a better frame of mind for answering questions or comprehending advice.

THE SEX FACTOR

Having an occasional attraction to one of your patients is normal. Remember, however, that you always must put the patient's welfare first. This means you must set aside your personal agenda, because your relationship with patients is primarily a fiduciary one. Consider getting help from a supervisor or therapist if you cannot separate your attraction from the care of your patient.

Sexualizing the relationship—endowing it with sexual significance, feelings, overtones, or behaviors—is dangerous, even if your patient seems to want or expect that type of behavior from you. It is your responsibility, not the patient's, to keep the relationship on a professional level.

When examining or treating patients, pay attention to where your hands are—both of them—so you can avoid unintended contact with sensitive areas. Pay attention, too, to where your eyes wander on your patients' bodies. Your gaze could be signalling that your main concern is not their health.

Flirting, sexual jokes, and innuendo all are very hazardous. If you are the one generating the flirting or innuendo, please stop. In some jurisdictions these may, in and of themselves, be held to constitute sexual misconduct. Moreover, even patients who appear to appreciate such behavior may just be trying to be polite; they actually may be put off by it. Some patients may be made so uncomfortable that they change doctors—with or without a single complaint to you. So if this is normal office behavior for you, consider revising your repertoire of office behavior.

If you have a patient who is acting in ways that would sexualize the relationship, don't just go along with the banter; try to set a more professional tone. Promptly record any unusual patient behavior in your notes, carefully documenting what occurred and how you handled the situation. This *may* give you some protection, should problems arise—and it *will* give you some warning, so that you can be alert and prepared at the patient's next visit.

— 17 —

The New Partnership

One of the best ways of avoiding the corruption of power is to share it.
—*Howard Brody,*
The Healer's Power, 1992

The doctor/patient relationship is undergoing a continuing process of transformation; it is moving from patriarchy toward partnership. All doctors and all patients need to assess their attitudes and behavior. Doctors need to rethink the way they practice, to accommodate patients who are becoming more like consumers. This isn't easy. But the results of adjusting to the new model of practice are well worth the effort it takes.

Many doctors are made uneasy by the prospect of sharing more information with their patients. They dread second-guessing and long debates.

But so far, those fears have failed to materialize. Patients do want more information from their doctors, but that is mostly so they can register a veto. "[In] one detailed study, only about 10% of patients said that they wanted information because they wished to participate substantially in their medical-care decisions."[1] And patients who are more involved, who have a greater understanding of what is being recommended and why, are markedly more likely to take prescribed medication and otherwise abide by treatment decisions.

Doctors who make the effort will be rewarded with better data for diagnosis and treatment, as their communication with patients improves. They will be relieved of some of their traditional burden of responsibility, as their patients take on more responsibility for their own care. They will be rewarded with a warmer, more collegial doctor/patient relationship

A true partnership between doctors and patients is just around the corner.

NOTE

1. Howard Brody, *The Healer's Power* (New Haven, Conn.: Yale University Press, 1992), 89.

Bibliography

Aburdene, Patricia, and John Naisbitt. *Megatrends for Women*. New York: Villard Books, 1992.

ACA Code of Ethics, 1994-1995. American Chiropractic Association, 1994.

Aronson, Stanley M. "The Perils of Sexual Ambiguity." Commentary. *The Providence Journal-Bulletin*, Monday, May 13, 1996, D-4.

Australian Medical Association, "Sexual Conduct Between Doctors and Their Patients: Position Statement—October 1994." As posted on the association's World Wide Web page, Australian Medical Association Limited, 1995.

Barlow, Janelle, and Claus Moller. *A Complaint Is a Gift*. San Francisco: Berrett-Koehler Publishers Inc., 1996.

Bell, Donald H. *Being a Man: The Paradox of Masculinity*. Lexington, Mass.: The Lewis Publishing Company, 1982.

Benjamin, Ben. "Bringing Boundaries to Bodywork." *Massage Therapy Journal*, 30(4) Winter 1991.

Benjamin, Ben. *Massage and Bodywork with Survivors of Abuse*. Medford, Mass.: Ben Benjamin, 1994.

Bernzweig, Jane, John I. Takayama, Ciaran Phibbs, Catherine Lewis, and Robert H. Pantell. "Gender Differences in Physician-Patient Communication: Evidence from Pediatric Visits." *Archives of Pediatrics & Adolescent Medicine*, 151 (June 1997): 586-591.

Bisbing, Steven B., Linda Mabus Jorgenson, and Pamela K. Sutherland. *Sexual Abuse by Professionals: A Legal Guide*. Charlottesville, Va.: *Michie*, 1995.

Bowers, Linda J. "Back to basics . . . The 'Slippery Slope': Boundary Issues for the Chiropractic Physician." *Topics in Clinical Chiropractic*, 1 (1994) 3: 1-8.

Bridges, Nancy A. "Meaning and Management of Attraction: Neglected Areas of Psychotherapy Training and Practice." *Psychotherapy*, 31 (Fall 1994) 3: 424-433.

Brody, Howard. *The Healer's Power*. New Haven, Conn.: Yale University Press, 1992.

Bryant, Anita. *The Anita Bryant Story: The Survival of Our Nation's Families and the*

Threat of Militant Homosexuality. Old Tappan, N.J.: Revell, 1977.

Bryant, Anita. Comments reported in *The New York Times*, June 5, 1977, 22.

Buchwald, Emilie, Pamela R. Fletcher, and Martha Roth, eds. *Transforming a Rape Culture.* Minneapolis, Minn.: Milkweed Editions, 1995.

Burbank, Victoria Katherine. *Fighting Women: Anger and Aggression in Aboriginal Australia.* Berkeley: University of California Press, 1994.

Campbell, Beatrice Stella (Mrs. Patrick Campbell), 1865-1940. Comments as reported in *The Duchess of Jermyn Street: The Life, Times and Good Times of Rosa Lewis of the Cavendish Hotel,* by Daphne Vivian Fielding (New York: Penguin Books, 1987), 37.

Caro, Wendy, and Angelica Redleaf. 1994 Survey of Licensing Boards in Mexico, Canada, the United States and the Caribbean. A study conducted for and distributed by the Federation of Chiropractic Licensing Boards (unpublished results).

Cassell, Joan. *Expected Miracles: Surgeons at Work.* Philadelphia: Temple University Press, 1991.

"Changing Medical Education: Let's Play Patient." *Consumer Reports,* 60 (February 1995): 83.

Colt, George Howe, with reporting by Anne Hollister. "The Magic of Touch: Massage's Healing Powers Make it Serious Medicine." *Life* (August 1997): 52-62.

DeLozier, James E., and Raymond O. Gagnon. National Ambulatory Medical Care Survey: 1989 Summary. Hyattsville, Md.: U.S. Department of Health and Human Services, Public Health Service, Centers for Disease Control, National Center for Health Statistics, 1991.

Disch, Estelle. "Are You in Trouble With a Client?" *Massage Therapy Journal,* 31(2) Summer 1992.

Dossey, Larry. "Medical Hexing: The Nocebo Effect and You." *Bottom Line/ Health,* June 1998, 15-16.

Edelstein, Lewis, translator. "The Hippocratic Oath." No. 1 of the *Supplements to the Bulletins of the History of Medicine.* Baltimore: Johns Hopkins University Press, 1943.

Ellis, Lee, and Linda Ebertz, eds. *Sexual Orientation: Toward Biological Understanding.* Westport, Conn.: Greenwood Publishing Group, Inc./Praeger Publishers, 1997.

Epstein, Cynthia Fuchs. *Women in Law.* Garden City, N.Y: Anchor Press/Doubleday, 1983.

Fielding, Daphne Vivian. *The Duchess of Jermyn Street: The Life, Times and Good Times of Rosa Lewis of the Cavendish Hotel.* New York: Penguin Books, 1987.

Freud, Sigmund. *On the Universal Tendency to Debasement in the Sphere of Love,* Section III. 1912.

Gabbard, Glen O. "Psychotherapists Who Transgress Sexual Boundaries With Patients." In *Breach of Trust: Sexual Exploitation by Health Care Professionals and Clergy,* John C. Gonsiorek, ed. Thousand Oaks, Calif.: Sage Publications, Inc., 1995, 133-144.

Gartrell, Nanette K., Nancy Milliken, William H. Goodson III, Sue Thiemann, and Bernard Lo. "Physician-Patient Sexual Contact: Prevalence and Problems." In *Breach of Trust: Sexual Exploitation by Health Care Professionals and Clergy,* John C. Gonsiorek, ed. Thousand Oaks, Calif.: Sage Publications, Inc., 1995,

18-28.

Gilligan, Carol. *In a Different Voice: Psychological Theory and Women's Development*. Boston: Harvard University Press, 1993.

Gonsiorek, John C. "Boundary Challenges When Both Therapist and Client Are Gay Males." In *Breach of Trust: Sexual Exploitation by Health Care Professionals and Clergy*, John C. Gonsiorek, ed. Thousand Oaks, Calif.: Sage Publications, Inc., 1995, 225-233.

Gonsiorek, John C., ed. *Breach of Trust: Sexual Exploitation by Health Care Professionals and Clergy*. Thousand Oaks, Calif.: Sage Publications, Inc., 1995.

Gonsiorek, John C. "Perpetrators." In *Breach of Trust: Sexual Exploitation by Health Care Professionals and Clergy*, John C. Gonsiorek, ed. Thousand Oaks, Calif.: Sage Publications, Inc., 1995, 129-131.

Gray, John. *Men are from Mars, Women are from Venus*. New York: HarperCollins, 1992.

Greenhouse, Linda. "Same-Sex Harassment Ruled Illegal." *The Providence Journal-Bulletin*, Tuesday, March 5, 1998, A-1.

Hall, J.A., R.H. Palmer, E.J. Orav, J.L. Hargraves, E.A. Wright, and A.T. Louis. "Performance, Quality, Gender and Professional Role: A Study of Physicians and Nonphysicians in Sixteen Ambulatory Care Practices." *Medical Care* (1990), 28: 489-501.

Handy, Bruce. "Deconstructing Leo: What the Men Don't Get, the Teen Girls Understand." *Time*, March 20, 1998, 53.

"The Happier the Doctor, the Better the Diagnosis, Study Finds." *The Providence Journal-Bulletin*, Feb. 23, 1995, A-4.

Helgesen, Sally. *The Female Advantage: Women's Ways of Leadership*. New York: Doubleday, 1990.

Herman, Judith Lewis. *Trauma and Recovery*. New York: BasicBooks, 1992.

Highway, Thomson. "It's Never O.K.: A Personal Viewpoint." Plenary address presented at *It's Never O.K., The Third International Conference on Sexual Exploitation by Health Professionals, Psychotherapists and Clergy*. Toronto, Ontario, Canada, Oct. 15, 1994.

Holm, Søren. "What Is Wrong With Compliance?" *Journal of Medical Ethics*, 19 (1993): 108-110.

Howatch, Susan. *Absolute Truths*. New York: Fawcett Crest, 1994.

"How Is Your Doctor Treating You?" *Consumer Reports*, 60 (February 1995), 81-88.

It's Never O.K., The Third International Conference on Sexual Exploitation by Health Professionals, Psychotherapists and Clergy, schedule and promotional materials for the conference, held in Toronto, Ontario, Canada, Oct. 13-15, 1994.

Jordan, Judith V. "The Movement of Mutuality and Power." Work in Progress No. 53. Wellesley, Mass.: The Stone Center for Developmental Services and Studies, Wellesley College, 1991.

Jorgenson, Linda Mabus. "Sexual Contact in Fiduciary Relationships: Legal Perspectives." In *Breach of Trust: Sexual Exploitation by Health Care Professionals and Clergy*, John C. Gonsiorek, ed. Thousand Oaks, Calif.: Sage Publications, Inc., 1995, 237-283.

Kaplan, Alexandra G. "Dichotomous Thought and Relational Processes in Therapy." Work in Progress No. 35. Wellesley, Mass.: The Stone Center for Developmental

Services and Studies, Wellesley College, 1988.

Kardener, Sheldon H., Marielle Fuller, and Ivan N. Mensh. "A Survey of Physicians' Attitudes and Practices Regarding Erotic and Nonerotic Contact with Patients." *American Journal of Psychiatry*, 130 (October 1973), 10, 1077-1081.

Kauth, Bill. *A Circle of Men: The Original Manual for Men's Support Groups*. New York: St. Martin's Press, 1992.

Keen, Sam. *Fire in the Belly: On Being a Man*. New York: Bantam Books, 1991.

Kimmel, Michael S. "Clarence, William, Iron Mike, Tailhook, Senator Packwook, Spur Posse, Magic . . . and Us." In *Transforming a Rape Culture*, Emilie Buchwald, Pamela R. Fletcher and Martha Roth, eds. Minneapolis, Minn.: Milkweed Editions, 1995, 119-138.

Kipnis, Aaron R. *Knights Without Armor: A Practical Guide for Men in the Quest of Masculine Soul*. Los Angeles, Calif.: St. Martin's Press, 1991.

Kitchner, K. "Dual Role Relationships: What Makes Them So Problematic?" *Journal of Counseling and Development*, 67 (1988), 217-221.

Kreuter, Matthew. Study produced by the Health Sciences Center, St. Louis University. St. Louis, Mo., 1995.

Kurtzig, Sandra. Comments as reported by Barbara Rudolph, in "Why Can't a Woman Manage More Like . . . a Woman?" *Time*, Special Issue, Women: The Road Ahead. 136 (1990), 53.

Leland, John. "Bisexuality is the wild card of our erotic life. Now it's coming out in the open—in pop culture, in cyberspace and on campus. But can you really have it both ways?" *Newsweek*, July 17, 1995, 44-50.

Margulis, Lynn, and Ann Dorion Sagan. *Mystery Dance on the Evolution of Human Sexuality*. New York: Summit Books, 1991.

McClintock, Martha K., and Kathleen Stern. "Regulation of Ovulation by Human Pheromones (Letter to *Nature*)." *Nature*, Vol. 392 (1998), 177.

Mead, Margaret. *Sex and Temperament in Three Primitive Societies*. New York: William Morrow and Company, 1935.

Miss Manners (columnist Judith Martin), "Sick of Doctors Testing Patience in Waiting Room." *The Providence Sunday Journal*, Feb. 26, 1995, H-6.

Montagu, Ashley. *Touching: The Human Significance of the Skin*. New York: Columbia University Press, 1971.

Morris, Desmond. *The Naked Ape: A Zoologist's Study of the Human Animal*. New York: McGraw-Hill, 1967.

Noël, Barbara, with Kathryn Watterson. *You Must Be Dreaming*. New York: Poseidon Press, 1992.

Northrup, Christiane. *Women's Wisdom, Women's Bodies: Creating Physical and Emotional Health and Healing*. New York: Bantam Books, 1995.

Papalia, Diane E., and Sally Wendkos Olds. *Psychology*, 2nd ed. New York: McGraw-Hill Book Company, 1985.

Prevention of Sexual Abuse of Patients: Introductory Instructor's Guide for Diploma Programs in Medical Radiation Technology. Toronto, Ontario, Canada: College of Medical Radiation Technologists of Ontario, 1994.

Prochaska, James O., and Wayne F. Velicer. "The Transtheoretical Model of Health Behavior Change." *American Journal of Health Promotion*, Sept. 1, 1997, 38.

Redleaf, Angelica. From the transcript of the keynote address, "Beneath the Surface:

A Deeper Look at Sexual Misconduct,'' delivered at the 62nd Annual Congress of the Federation of Chiropractic Licensing Boards, in Portland, Ore., May 11, 1995. Warwick, R.I.: Association for Chiropractic Excellence, Inc., 1995.

Roberts-Henry, Melissa. "Criminalization in Colorado: Overview and Opinion." In *Breach of Trust: Sexual Exploitation by Health Care Professionals and Clergy,* John C. Gonsiorek, ed. Thousand Oaks, Calif.: Sage Publications, Inc., 1995, 338-347.

Robinson, Gail E., Rachel Edney, Joan Bishop, and Stella Blackshaw. "Preventing Sexual Exploitation in Doctor-Patient Relationships through Medical Training." A conference session at *It's Never O.K., The Third International Conference on Sexual Exploitation by Health Professionals, Psychotherapists and Clergy.* Toronto, Ontario, Canada, Oct. 14, 1994.

Roter, Debra L., and Judith A. Hall. *Doctors Talking with Patients/Patients Talking with Doctors: Improving Communication in Medical Visits.* Westport, Conn.: Auburn House, 1992.

Rudolph, Barbara. "Why Can't a Woman Manage More Like . . . a Woman?" *Time,* Vol. 136: Special Issue 53, Fall 1990.

Schoener, Gary R. "Employer/Supervisor Liability and Risk Management: An Administrator's View." In *Breach of Trust: Sexual Exploitation by Health Care Professionals and Clergy,* John C. Gonsiorek, ed. Thousand Oaks, Calif.: Sage Publications, Inc., 1995, 300-311.

Schoener, Gary R. From a private telephone conversation in November 1994.

Schoener, Gary R. "Historical Overview." In *Breach of Trust: Sexual Exploitation by Health Care Professionals and Clergy,* John C. Gonsiorek, ed. Thousand Oaks, Calif.: Sage Publications, Inc., 1995, 3-17.

Schoener, Gary R., and John C. Gonsiorek. "Assessment, Treatment and Supervision of the Professional Offender." A pre-conference seminar at *It's Never O.K., The Third International Conference on Sexual Exploitation by Health* Professionals, Psychotherapists and Clergy. Toronto, Ontario, Canada, Oct. 13, 1994.

"Sexual Harassment in the Workplace: Corporate Strategies for Protection and Defense." Seminar handout. Providence, R.I.: Licht & Semonoff, Attorneys at Law, May 2, 1995.

The Sexuality Information and Education Council of the United States. *SIECUS Conference on Religion and Sexuality and Human Values.* New York: Association Press, 1974.

Sheehy, Gail. *New Passages: Mapping Your Life Across Time.* New York: Random House, 1995.

Spicer, Larry A. From the outline for his address "Professional Boundaries for the Federation of Chiropractic Licensing Boards," which was delivered at the 62nd Annual Congress of the Federation of Chiropractic Licensing Boards, in Portland, Ore., in May 1995. Minnesota: Larry A. Spicer, April 1996.

Stahl, Michael J., and Stephen M. Foreman. *Sexual Misconduct: Ethical, Clinical and Legal Ramifications for the Chiropractic Profession.* Des Moines, Iowa: NCMIC Insurance Co., 1997.

Steinem, Gloria. *Revolution from Within: A Book of Self-Esteem.* Boston: Little, Brown and Company, 1992.

"Tangled Case of Sexual Molestation Pits a Doctor Against 8 Poor Women." *The New*

York Times, National Ed., Jan. 29, 1995, 18.

Tannahill, Reay. *Sex In History*. Chelsea, Miss.: Scarborough House, 1992.

Tannen, Deborah. *Talking from 9 to 5: How Women's and Men's Conversational Styles Affect Who Gets Heard, Who Gets Credit, and What Gets Done at Work.* New York: William Morrow and Company, 1994.

Tannen, Deborah. *You Just Don't Understand: Women and Men in Conversation.* New York: Ballantine Books, 1990.

Taylor, J. Lionel. Excerpt from his landmark book, *The Stages of Human Life*, as quoted in *Touching: The Human Significance of the Skin*, by Ashley Montagu. New York: Columbia University Press, 1971.

Tiger, Lionel. *Men in Groups*. New York: Random House, 1969.

Toufexis, Anastasia. "Coming from a Different Place: Men and Women Just Don't See Things the Same Way. Some Surprising New Studies of Schoolgirls Show Why." *Time*, Special Issue, Women: The Road Ahead, 136, No. 19 (Fall 1990), 64-66.

Twaddle, Andrew C. *A Sociology of Health*. Saint Louis: Mosby, 1977.

Yanity, Kathleen. "Schwarzkopf Talks Leadership; His Advice: 'When Placed in Command, Take Charge.' " *The Providence Journal-Bulletin*, Friday, March 20, 1998, F-1.

Yarnold, P.R., *et al.* "Androgeny Predicts Empathy for Trainees in Medicine." *Perceptual Motor Skills*, 77 (October 1993): 576-578.

Recommended Reading

Allen, Tim. *Don't Stand Too Close to a Naked Man*. New York: Hyperion, 1994. A humorous compilation of autobiographical material, plus commentary on sexuality and gender roles in modern society, from the star of the popular television series *Home Improvement*.

Ashcraft, Norman, and Albert E. Scheffen. *People Space: The Making and Breaking of Human Boundaries*. Garden City, N.Y., 1976.

Barlow, Janelle, and Claus Moller. *A Complaint Is a Gift*. San Francisco: Berrett-Koehler Publishers Inc., 1996.

Baron, Dennis. *Grammar and Gender*. New Haven: Yale University Press, 1986.

Bell, Donald H. *Being a Man: The Paradox of Masculinity*. Lexington, Mass.: The Lewis Publishing Company, 1982.

Benjamin, Ben. *Massage and Bodywork with Survivors of Abuse*. Medford, Mass.: Ben Benjamin, 1994.

Bisbing, Steven B., Linda Mabus Jorgenson, and Pamela K. Sutherland. *Sexual Abuse by Professionals: A Legal Guide*. Charlottesville, Va.: *Michie*, 1995.

Brody, Howard. *The Healer's Power*. New Haven, Conn.: Yale University Press, 1992.

Brothers, Joyce. *What Every Woman Should Know About Men*. New York: Simon & Schuster, 1981.

Buchwald, Emilie, Pamela R. Fletcher, and Martha Roth, eds. *Transforming a Rape Culture*. Minneapolis, Minn.: Milkweed Editions, 1995.

Cassell, Joan. *Expected Miracles: Surgeons at Work*. Philadelphia: Temple University Press, 1991.

"Changing Medical Education: Let's Play Patient." *Consumer Reports*, 60 (February 1995): 83.

Colt, George Howe, with reporting by Anne Hollister. "The Magic of Touch: Massage's Healing Powers Make it Serious Medicine." *Life* (August 1997): 52-62.

Coontz, Stephanie. *The Way We Really Are: Coming to Terms with America's Changing Families*. New York: Harper Collins Publishers, Inc./Basic Books, 1997.

Ellis, Lee, and Linda Ebertz, Eds. *Sexual Orientation: Toward Biological Understanding*. Westport, Conn.: Greenwood Publishing Group, Inc./Praeger Publishers, 1997.

Gilligan, Carol. *In a Different Voice: Psychological Theory and Women's Development*. Boston: Harvard University Press, 1993.
Gonsiorek, John C., ed. *Breach of Trust: Sexual Exploitation by Health Care Professionals and Clergy*. Thousand Oaks, Calif.: Sage Publications, Inc., 1995.

Helgesen, Sally. *The Female Advantage: Women's Ways of Leadership*. New York: Doubleday, 1990.
Herman, Judith Lewis. *Trauma and Recovery*. New York: BasicBooks, 1992.
Heyward, Carter. *When Boundaries Betray Us: Beyond Illusions of What is Ethical in Therapy and Life*. HarperSanFrancisco, a Division of HarperCollins Publishers, 1994. Heyward, an Episcopal priest, ethicist, and professor of theology, writes about her own experience as a patient in psychotherapy of being traumatized, not by the breaking of boundaries, but by their too-rigid observance and the withholding of emotional ties.
Holm, Søren. "What Is Wrong with Compliance?" *Journal of Medical Ethics*, 19 (1993): 108-110.

Jordan, Judith V. "The Movement of Mutuality and Power." Work in Progress No. 53. Wellesley, Mass.: The Stone Center for Developmental Services and Studies, Wellesley College, 1991.

Kardener, Sheldon H., Marielle Fuller, and Ivan N. Mensh. "A Survey of Physicians' Attitudes and Practices Regarding Erotic and Nonerotic Contact with Patients." *American Journal of Psychiatry*, 130 (October 1973), 10, 1077-1081.
Kauth, Bill. *A Circle of Men: The Original Manual for Men's Support Groups*. New York: St. Martin's Press, 1992.
Keen, Sam. *Fire in the Belly: On Being a Man*. New York: Bantam Books, 1991.

Loustauna, Martha O., and Elisa J. Sobo. *The Cultural Context of Health, Illness, and Medicine*. Westport, Conn.: Greenwood Publishing Group, Inc./Bergin & Garvey, 1998.

Margulis, Lynn, and Ann Dorion Sagan. *Mystery Dance on the Evolution of Human Sexuality*. New York: Summit Books, 1991.
Montagu, Ashley. *Touching: The Human Significance of the Skin*. New York: Columbia University Press, 1971.
Morris, Desmond. *The Naked Ape: A Zoologist's Study of the Human Animal*. New York: McGraw-Hill, 1967.

Noël, Barbara, with Kathryn Watterson. *You Must Be Dreaming*. New York: Poseidon

Press, 1992.

Northrup, Christiane. *Women's Wisdom, Women's Bodies: Creating Physical and Emotional Health and Healing*. New York: Bantam Books, 1995.

Phipps, William E. *Assertive Biblical Women*. Westport, Conn.: Greenwood Publishing Group, Inc./Greenwood Press, 1992.

Prevention of Sexual Abuse of Patients: Introductory Instructor's Guide for Diploma Programs in Medical Radiation Technology. Toronto, Ontario, Canada: College of Medical Radiation Technologists of Ontario, 1994.

Prochaska, James O., and Wayne F. Velicer. "The Transtheoretical Model of Health Behavior Change." *American Journal of Health Promotion*, Sept. 1, 1997, 38.

Rabin, Susan, with Barbara Lagowski. *How to Attract Anyone, Anytime, Anyplace: The Smart Guide to Flirting*. New York: Plume, an imprint of Dutton Signet, a division of Penguin Books USA, Inc., 1993. More than just a how-not-to book, this slender paperback also is crammed full of easy-to-understand descriptions of body language and conversational styles.

Roter, Debra L., and Judith A. Hall. *Doctors Talking with Patients/Patients Talking with Doctors: Improving Communication in Medical Visits*. Westport, Conn.: Auburn House, 1992.

Schwartz, M.A. *Listen to Me, Doctor: Taking Charge of Your Own Health Care*. Aspen: MacMurray & Beck, 1995.

Stahl, Michael J., and Stephen M. Foreman. *Sexual Misconduct: Ethical, Clinical and Legal Ramifications for the Chiropractic Profession*. Des Moines, Iowa: NCMIC Insurance Co., 1997.

Sutherland, Pamela K. *Sexual Abuse by Therapists, Physicians, Attorneys, and Other Professionals*. World Wide Web (posted at http://wwlia.org/us-prosx.htm): Pamela K. Sutherland and the World Wide Legal Information Association (WWLIA), 1996.

"Tangled Case of Sexual Molestation Pits a Doctor Against 8 Poor Women." *The New York Times*, National Ed., Jan. 29, 1995, 18.

Tannahill, Reay. *Sex In History*. Chelsea, Miss.: Scarborough House, 1992.

Tannen, Deborah. *Talking from 9 to 5: How Women's and Men's Conversational Styles Affect Who Gets Heard, Who Gets Credit, and What Gets Done at Work*. New York: William Morrow and Company, 1994.

Tannen, Deborah. *You Just Don't Understand: Women and Men in Conversation*. New York: Ballantine Books, 1990.

Tiger, Lionel. *Men in Groups*. New York: Random House, 1969.

Toufexis, Anastasia. "Coming from a Different Place: Men and Women Just Don't See Things the Same Way. Some Surprising New Studies of Schoolgirls Show Why." *Time*, Special Issue, Women: The Road Ahead, 136, No. 19 (Fall 1990), 64-66.

Wood, Elizabeth J., and Floris W. Wood. *She Said, He Said: What Men and Women Really Think About Money, Sex, Politics and Other Issues of Essence*. Detroit: Visible Ink Press, 1992.

Recommended Viewing

Article 99 (U.S.: Orion, 1991), with Ray Liotta and Kiefer Sutherland. Howard Deutch's lighthearted drama about doctors at a V.A. hospital, who battle the bureaucracy on behalf of their patients.

Awakenings (U.S.: RCA/Columbia, 1990), with Robert DeNiro and Robin Williams. Penny Marshall's drama about a comatose patient and the doctor who refuses to give up on him—and, eventually, helps the patient to regain consciousness after 30 years in a coma. Based on Dr. Oliver Sacks's book and real-life experiences.

Boxing Helena (U.S.: Mainline Pictures, 1993), with Julian Sands and Sherilyn Fenn. Harrowing drama about a doctor's fantasy of taking possession—surgically—of the woman he loves, so that she can't leave him.

City of Joy (England/France: 1992), with Patrick Swayze and Pauline Collins. Roland Jaffe's drama about a doctor's quest for self-knowledge in the slums of Calcutta, in which he finds joy and satisfaction by learning to practice—and to live—for the sake of his patients rather than for himself. (Selflessness this extreme is required of saints, not doctors, but this film still does a good job of illustrating the difference between serving one's own needs and serving the needs of the patient.) The screenplay, by Mark Medoff, is based on Dominique Lapier's book.

Compromising Positions (U.S.: 1985), with Susan Sarandon, Raul Julia, and Joe Mantegna. Frank Perry's mystery/black comedy about a periodontist who engages in abusive, sexually inappropriate behavior with many of his female patients, and about the search for his murderer. Based on the novel by Susan Isaacs, who also wrote the screenplay.

Dad (U.S.: 1989), with Ted Danson, Jack Lemmon, and Olympia Dukakis. Gary David Goldberg's drama about a father's fatal illness and about the attempts of him and his adult son to come to terms with each other and the health-care system.

Dead Ringers (Canada: 1988), with Jeremy Irons and Genevieve Bujold. David Cronenberg's drama about twin gynecologists in joint practice, who share their patients and their lovers; and about the choice one of them is forced to make, when he must decide whether to report his twin. Based on a true story.

Doc Hollywood (U.S.: 1991), with Michael J. Fox and Julie Warner. Michael Canton-Jones's comedy about a young doctor *en route* to Los Angeles, to take up a career in plastic surgery, who learns—after his car breaks down in a small town that has been unable to attract a new doctor, and the townsfolk try to keep him there—that there is more to a practice and to life than the big bucks and fast cars that he had been looking for when he went to medical school.

The Doctor (U.S.: 1991), with Elizabeth Perkins, Mandy Patinkin, William Hurt, and Christine Lahti. Ronda Haines's drama about a successful but stand-offish surgeon who develops throat cancer and learns what it's like to be a patient. Based on Dr. Ed Rosenbaum's true story, as described in the book *A Taste of My Own Medicine*.

Everything You Always Wanted to Know About Sex (But Were Afraid to Ask) (U.S.: 1972), with Woody Allen, John Carradine, Lou Jacobi, Louise Lasser, Tony Randall, Lynn Redgrave and Burt Reynolds. Woody Allen's comedy about contemporary attitudes toward sexuality and reproduction; it includes an amusing doctor/patient scene. Distantly related to the self-help book of the same name.

Gross Anatomy (U.S.: 1989), with Matthew Modine, Daphne Zuniga, and Christine Lahti. Thom Eberhardt's black comedy about medical students learning the ropes; it features exaggerated and easy-to-recognize depictions of common doctor and patient roles. The Oscar-winning screenplay is by Paddy Chayevsky.

The Hospital (U.S.: 1971), with George C. Scott and Diana Rigg. Arthur Hiller's drama about a discouraged doctor's unique relationship with a troubled patient.

King of the Gypsies (U.S.: 1978), with Eric Roberts, Judd Hirsch, Susan Sarandon, Brooke Shields, Annie Potts, Shelley Winters, David Grisman, and Stephan Grappelli. Frank Pierson's drama about three generations of gypsies in New York City. The scenes of the gypsy "king" in the hospital illustrate the complications that can arise when dealing with patients of a different ethnic or cultural background.

Little Shop of Horrors (U.S.: 1986), with Rick Moranis, Ellen Greene, Vincent Gardenia, Steve Martin, James Belushi, and John Candy. Frank Oz's musical black comedy about a curio shop and the owner's carnivorous plant, Audrey II. Watch for Steve Martin's over-the-top portrayal of the dentist, whose highly inappropriate style of practice is designed to fulfill his needs, not those of his patients.

Lorenzo's Oil (U.S.: 1993), with Nick Nolte, Susan Sarandon, and Peter Ustinov. Drama about the parents of a boy with a rare genetic illness, who nudge and use and circumvent the health-care system in their efforts to find an effective treatment for their son.

Man Facing Southwest (Argentina: 1986), with Hugo Sato, Lorenzo Quinteros, and Ines Vernengo. Eliseo Subiela's drama about the relationship between an asylum inmate with unusual powers and his psychiatrist. This intense art-house film is in Spanish, but is available with English subtitles.

The New Interns (U.S.: 1964), with Michael Callan, Dean Jones, Telly Salvalas, Inger Stevens, George Segal, and Barbara Eden. John Rich directs this critically acclaimed sequel to the hospital soap-opera *The Interns*.

Plague (Canada: 1978), with Daniel Pilon, Kate Reid, and Celine Lomez. Ed Hunt's existential drama about an outbreak of the bubonic plague.

Resurrection (U.S.: 1980), with Ellen Burstyn and Sam Shepard. Daniel Petrie's drama about a woman who emerges from a coma after an automobile accident to find that she now has remarkable healing powers; it deals peripherally with the medical establishment.

Vital Signs (U.S.:   1990), with Adrian Pasdar, Diane Lane, Jimmy Smits. Marisa Silver's drama about third-year medical students shows them doing rounds, questioning authority, competing with one another, and learning to assume the doctor role.

Wild Strawberries (Sweden: 1957), with Victor Sjostrom, Ingrid Thulin, and Bibi Anderson. The classic Ingmar Bergman drama about an aging doctor in Stockholm, looking back on the achievements and disappointments of a lifetime.

Young Dr. Kildare (U.S.:   1938), with Lew Ayers, Lionel Barrymore, and Lynne Carver. The first episode in the MGM series, directed by Harold S. Burquet, this film shows Kildare as a young med-school graduate who must decide whether to become a big-city doctor at Blair General Hospital or a small-town doctor in his father's practice.

Young Doctors in Love (U.S.:   1982), Michael McKean, Sean Young, Harry Dean Stanton, and a host of others in cameo roles, among them, Demi Moore. Garry Marshall's comedy has little plot, but lots of jokes, many of which illuminate the doctor role.

Index

About the Authors

ANGELICA REDLEAF, D.C.

Angelica Redleaf is the president of Redleaf Wellness Center, Inc., a private chiropractic practice in Providence, R.I. She also is founder and president of SafeCare, Inc., and past president of the Association for Chiropractic Excellence, or ACE.

A practicing chiropractor since 1978, Dr. Redleaf has served as president, vice president, secretary, and as a member of the Board of Governors for the chiropractic society in her home state of Rhode Island.

Since 1992, she also has been a provider of educational and consulting services to professional societies, state licensing boards and individual doctors. Her unique vision of the changing doctor/patient relationship is the basis of her practice-building and practice-protection services.

She is a member of the post-graduate faculty at New York Chiropractic College, where she earned her Doctor of Chiropractic degree. She earned her baccalaureate at Hunter College, in education and anthropology. Her background includes teaching, social work, and studies in psychology.

SUSAN A. BAIRD

Susan Baird is a copy editor and sometime special-assignment reporter at *The Providence Journal*, in Providence, R.I., and also works as a free-lance writer, editor, and computer consultant. She previously was the managing editor of the *Kent County Daily Times*, in West Warwick, R.I. Before venturing into journalism, she was a published biochemist, working as a research assistant at the Harvard School of Dental Medicine, Brown University, and the University of Rhode Island, where she was a member of the volunteer ambulance corps.

ISBN 0-86569-285-8

90000>

EAN

9 780865 692855

HARDCOVER BAR CODE